GROW

Natural Remedies From *100* Herbs

∎∎∎∎∎∎∎∎∎∎∎

Herbal Book for Beginners

For everyone venturing into the world of herbal remedies, this book is dedicated to you! It's our sincere hope that planting, growing and harvesting your own herbs will help you on your way towards natural well-being, and enables you to take control of your personal health from this day forward. In this book, discover the knowledge, inspiration, peace, and health that we all strive for.

The Lush Grove

"Grow Medicine, Natural Remedies from 100 Herbs" provides information on cultivating and using herbal remedies for wellness purposes. It is intended for educational purposes only and should not be considered medical advice. The use of herbs and natural remedies should complement, not replace, professional medical advice, diagnosis, or treatment. Always consult with a healthcare professional before starting any new health regimen, especially if you have pre-existing conditions or are taking medication.

Join Our Lush Grove Community

(the-lush-grove-home.carrd.co)

Unlock Exclusive Content

Choose your FREE welcome gift

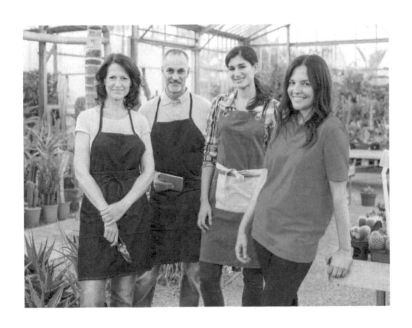

Plant Photo Samples

600 Color Images
(6 per each plant)

Join this growing book!

In Chapter 12, each of the 100 individual plants is accompanied by a QR code that directs you to a webpage with color photo samples. The first six pictures on the webpage are provided by us, while the rest are contributions from readers like you!

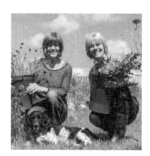 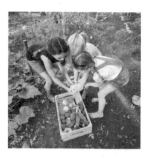 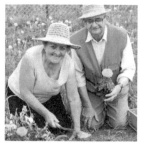

We invite you to email us photos of any of the 100 plants you are currently growing or using, along with a brief description of what we're seeing in your photo. Your contributions will be featured on the unique webpage dedicated to each plant in this Growing Book!

Top 100 Herbs to Grow

Aloe Vera, 89
Angelica, 92
Anise, 95
Ashwagandha, 98
Astragalus, 101
Basil, 104
Bay Leaf, 108
Bee Balm, 111
Bergamot, 116
Burdock, 120
Calendula, 123
Caraway, 127
Cardamom, 130
Catnip, 134
Cat's Claw, 138
Chamomile, 142
Chaste Tree, 145
Chicory, 148
Chives, 152
Cilantro, 155
Cinnamon, 159
Clove, 163
Cumin, 167
Damiana, 170
Dandelion, 174
Dong Quai, 178
Echinacea, 182
Elderberry, 186
Elecampane, 189
Eucalyptus, 193
Fennel, 196
Fenugreek, 200
Feverfew, 204
Garlic, 207
Ginger, 211
Ginkgo Biloba, 214
Ginseng, 218

Goldenseal, 222
Gotu Kola, 226
Hawthorn, 229
Holy Basil, 232
Hops, 236
Horehound, 240
Horsetail, 244
Hyssop, 247
Lady's Mantle, 251
Lavender, 254
Lemon Balm, 258
Lemon Verbena, 262
Lemongrass, 265
Licorice, 268
Lovage, 272
Maca, 275
Marjoram, 278
Marshmallow Root, 282
Meadowsweet, 285
Milk Thistle, 288
Mint, 291
Motherwort, 295
Mullein, 298
Neem, 301
Nettle, 304
Nutmeg, 308
Oregano, 312
Parsley, 316
Passionflower, 319
Peppermint, 322
Perilla, 327
Plantain, 330
Purslane, 334

Raspberry Leaf, 338
Red Clover, 341
Rhodiola Rosea, 344
Rosehip, 347
Rosemary, 351
Saffron, 355
Sage, 358
Schisandra, 361
Shepherd's Purse, 364
Skullcap, 367
Slippery Elm, 370
Soapwort, 373
Sorrel, 376
Spearmint, 379
Spikenard, 383
Stevia, 386
St. John's Wort, 389
Sweet Woodruff, 392
Tarragon, 395
Thyme, 398
Turmeric, 402
Uva Ursi, 406
Valerian, 409
Vervain, 412
Watercress, 416
White Willow Bark, 420
Wild Yam, 423
Witch Hazel, 426
Yarrow, 429
Yucca, 433

Our Body's 12 Major Systems

The Digestive System

Aloe Vera, Angelica, Anise, Basil, Calendula, Cardamom, Chamomile, Chicory, Cinnamon, Clove, Dandelion, Fennel, Fenugreek, Garlic, Ginger, Licorice, Marshmallow Root, Milk Thistle, Mint, Peppermint, Plantain, Slippery Elm, Tarragon, Turmeric.

The Nervous System

Ashwagandha, Basil, Bee Balm, Bergamot, Catnip, Chamomile, Damiana, Ginkgo Biloba, Gotu Kola, Hops, Lavender, Lemon Balm, Lemon Verbena, Licorice, Passionflower, Peppermint, Rhodiola Rosea, Sage, Skullcap, St. John's Wort, Valerian, Wild Yam.

The Respiratory System

Angelica, Anise, Bee Balm, Echinacea, Elderberry, Elecampane, Fennel, Garlic, Ginger, Horehound, Hyssop, Lavender, Lemon Balm, Licorice, Marshmallow Root, Mullein, Peppermint, Plantain, Sage, Thyme, Yarrow.

The Cardiovascular System

Aloe Vera, Angelica, Ashwagandha, Astragalus, Garlic, Ginkgo Biloba, Goldenseal, Gotu Kola, Hawthorn, Holy Basil, Horsetail, Lemon Balm, Motherwort, Rosemary, Sage, Thyme, Turmeric, Yarrow.

The Skin and Integumentary System (Hair, Nails, and Glands)

Aloe Vera, Basil, Bee Balm, Bergamot, Burdock, Calendula, Chamomile, Dandelion, Echinacea, Elderberry, Fenugreek, Gotu Kola, Lavender, Lemon Balm, Licorice, Marshmallow Root, Neem, Nettle, Plantain, Red Clover, Rosemary, Sage, St. John's Wort, Turmeric, Witch Hazel, Yarrow.

The Immune System

Aloe Vera, Astragalus, Basil, Bee Balm, Calendula, Catnip, Echinacea, Elderberry, Garlic, Ginger, Goldenseal, Holy Basil, Lemon Balm, Licorice, Neem, Oregano, Rosemary, Sage, Schisandra, Thyme, Turmeric, Uva Ursi, Yarrow.

The Urinary System

Burdock, Dandelion, Marshmallow Root, Nettle, Parsley, Uva Ursi, Yarrow.

The Muscular System

Arnica, Ashwagandha, Chamomile, Comfrey, Ginger, Gotu Kola, Lavender, Lemongrass, Rosemary, Sage, St. John's Wort, Turmeric, Valerian, Yarrow.

The Skeletal System

Dandelion, Horsetail, Nettle, Red Clover, Turmeric, White Willow Bark.

The Reproductive System

Angelica, Anise, Ashwagandha, Borage, Chaste Tree, Damiana, Dong Quai, Fenugreek, Ginger, Gotu Kola, Hawthorn, Lady's Mantle, Lavender, Lemon Balm, Licorice, Motherwort, Raspberry Leaf, Red Clover, Rosemary, Sage, Schisandra, Skullcap, St. John's Wort, Valerian, Wild Yam, Yarrow.

The Endocrine System

Ashwagandha, Chaste Tree, Dong Quai, Fenugreek, Holy Basil, Licorice, Rhodiola Rosea, Sage, Schisandra, Wild Yam.

The Lymphatic System

Astragalus, Calendula, Dandelion, Echinacea, Elderberry, Goldenseal, Mullein, Red Clover, Yarrow.

A Few Herbal Applications

(Specifics on how to grow and use each herb in Chapter 12)

Acid Reflux - Slippery Elm, 370

Acne Treatment - Neem, 301; Witch Hazel, 426; Lavender, 254

Adrenal Cortex Support - Licorice, 268; Holy Basil, 232

Adrenal Health - Ashwagandha, 98; Holy Basil, 232; Licorice, 268

Adrenal Tumor Management - Licorice, 268; Holy Basil, 232

Allergy Relief - Nettle, 304

Alzheimer's Prevention - Ginkgo Biloba, 214; Turmeric, 402

Anti-aging - Lavender, 254; Rosemary, 351; Rosehip, 347

Anti-inflammatory - Arnica; Chamomile, 142; Lavender, 254; Turmeric, 402; Ginger, 211; Chamomile, 142

Anti-itch - Peppermint, 322; Calendula, 123

Antibacterial Health - Garlic, 207; Thyme, 398

Antifungal - Garlic, 207; Oregano, 312; Thyme, 398

Antioxidant Support - Elderberry, 186; Turmeric, 402; Ginger, 211; Nettle, 304; Milk Thistle, 288; Rosemary, 351; Thyme, 398; Sage, 358

Antiseptic - Thyme, 398; Witch Hazel, 426; Yarrow, 429

Antiviral Help - Echinacea, 182; Elderberry, 186; Lemon Balm, 258

Anxiety - Chamomile, 142; Lavender, 254

Appetite Support - Angelica, 92

Arrhythmia - Hawthorn, 229; Motherwort, 295

Arteries Health - Garlic, 207; Ginger, 211; Hawthorn, 229

Arthritic (anti) - Nettle, 304; Burdock, 120; Yucca, 433

Arthritis - Turmeric, 402; Ginger, 211; Yucca, 433

Asthma - Hyssop, 247; Mullein, 298

Atherosclerosis - Garlic, 207; Hawthorn, 229; Turmeric, 402

Autoimmune Regulation - Ashwagandha, 98; Astragalus, 101; Licorice, 268

Autoimmune Thyroid Management - Ashwagandha, 98

Bacterial Infections - Echinacea, 182; Garlic, 207; Thyme, 398

Bile Production - Dandelion, 174; Milk Thistle, 288

Bladder Support - Horsetail, 244

Bloating - Fennel, 196; Peppermint, 322

Blood Cell Support - Nettle, 304; Dandelion, 174

Blood Clot Prevention - Garlic, 207; Ginkgo Biloba, 214; Turmeric, 402

Blood Pressure - Garlic, 207; Hawthorn, 229

Blood Purification - Burdock, 120; Dandelion, 174; Red Clover, 341; Nettle, 304

Blood Sugar Regulation - Cinnamon, 159; Fenugreek, 200

Blood Vessels Health - Hawthorn, 229; Ginkgo Biloba, 214; Garlic, 207

Bone Density Support - Horsetail, 244; Red Clover, 341; Nettle, 304

Brain Health - Ginkgo Biloba, 214; Ashwagandha, 98

Breast Health - Red Clover, 341; Fenugreek, 200

Breathing Capacity - Mullein, 298

Bronchial Tubes - Anise, 95; Hyssop, 247; Thyme, 398

Burn Relief - Aloe Vera, 89; Lavender, 254; Calendula, 123

Calcium Absorption - Nettle, 304; Horsetail, 244; Red Clover, 341

Cardiac Anxiety - Lavender, 254; Lemon Balm, 258

Cardiac Tonic - Hawthorn, 229; Rosemary, 351; Motherwort, 295

Cardiovascular Strength - Astragalus, 101; Hawthorn, 229

Cartilage Repair - Turmeric, 402; Ginger, 211

Cellular Support - Astragalus, 101; Schisandra, 361

Cervical Wellness - Echinacea, 182; Goldenseal, 222; Garlic, 207

Cholesterol Health - Garlic, 207

Chronic Pain - Arnica; St. John's Wort, 389

Circulation Boost - Ginkgo Biloba, 214; Ginger, 211; Hawthorn, 229

Circulation Improvement - Ginkgo Biloba, 214; Ginger, 211

Cognitive Function - Ginkgo Biloba, 214; Gotu Kola, 226

Cold Sores - Lemon Balm, 258; Echinacea, 182; Licorice, 268

Collagen Production - Gotu Kola, 226; Horsetail, 244; Aloe Vera, 89

Colon Health - Dandelion, 174

Concentration - Ginkgo Biloba, 214; Rosemary, 351

Constipation - Aloe Vera, 89

COPD - Thyme, 398; Licorice, 268

Cortisol Reduction - Holy Basil, 232; Ashwagandha, 98; Rhodiola Rosea, 344

Cough - Horehound, 240; Hyssop, 247; Licorice, 268; Mullein, 298; Thyme, 398

Cramps - Chamomile, 142; Ginger, 211

Dementia - Ginkgo Biloba, 214; Ashwagandha, 98; Rosemary, 351

Depression - St. John's Wort, 389; Lemon Balm, 258

Detox - Dandelion, 174; Red Clover, 341; Milk Thistle, 288; Nettle, 304

Diabetes - Cinnamon, 159; Fenugreek, 200

Diarrhea - Chamomile, 142; Slippery Elm, 370

Digestive Support - Chamomile, 142; Ginger, 211; Peppermint, 322; Licorice, 268; Basil, 104

Digestive Tract - Licorice, 268; Aloe Vera, 89

Diuretic Support - Dandelion, 174; Parsley, 316; Nettle, 304; Horsetail, 244

Ear Infections - Garlic, 207; Mullein, 298; Echinacea, 182

Eczema Relief - Chamomile, 142; Licorice, 268; Calendula, 123

Edema Treatment - Dandelion, 174; Parsley, 316

Emotional Balance - St. John's Wort, 389; Lemon Balm, 258

Endocrine Balancer - Ashwagandha, 98; Holy Basil, 232; Licorice, 268

Endocrine Disruptor Detoxification - Milk Thistle, 288; Dandelion, 174

Endocrine Inflammation - Turmeric, 402; Ginger, 211

Endocrine Support - Ashwagandha, 98; Holy Basil, 232; Licorice, 268

Endocrine Tumors - Turmeric, 402

Endometrial Health - Turmeric, 402; Milk Thistle, 288

Endothelial Health - Ginkgo Biloba, 214; Garlic, 207

Energy Boost - Ashwagandha, 98; Rhodiola Rosea, 344

Esophagus Health - Slippery Elm, 370; Licorice, 268

Estrogen Balance - Red Clover, 341

Eye Health, Vision - Ginkgo Biloba, 214

Fatigue - Ginseng, 218; Ashwagandha, 98; Rhodiola Rosea, 344

Fertility Support - Red Clover, 341; Raspberry Leaf, 338; Ashwagandha, 98; Damiana, 170

Fibromyalgia - St. John's Wort, 389; Ashwagandha, 98; Turmeric, 402

Flatulence Reduction - Nutmeg, 308

Flu - Echinacea, 182; Elderberry, 186; Ginger, 211; Yarrow, 429

Focus - Ginkgo Biloba, 214; Rosemary, 351

Fracture Healing - Horsetail, 244

Fungal (anti) - Oregano, 312; Garlic, 207

Fungal Infections - Garlic, 207; Thyme, 398

Gallbladder Health - Milk Thistle, 288

Gas - Anise, 95; Fennel, 196

Gastric Health - Licorice, 268; Marshmallow Root, 282

Gastrointestinal Help - Aloe Vera, 89; Slippery Elm, 370

GERD - Slippery Elm, 370; Marshmallow Root, 282; Licorice, 268

Gum Health - Clove, 163; Chamomile, 142; Echinacea, 182

Gut Health - Slippery Elm, 370; Marshmallow Root, 282

Gut Inflammation - Aloe Vera, 89; Turmeric, 402

Hair Follicles - Horsetail, 244

Headache - Feverfew, 204; Peppermint, 322

Heart Health - Hawthorn, 229; Motherwort, 295; Garlic, 207; Rosemary, 351

Heart Palpitations - Motherwort, 295; Lemon Balm, 258; Hawthorn, 229

Heartburn Relief - Licorice, 268; Slippery Elm, 370

Hemorrhoids - Witch Hazel, 426; Yarrow, 429

Hepatitis - Milk Thistle, 288; Dandelion, 174; Schisandra, 361

Herpes - Lemon Balm, 258; Echinacea, 182; Licorice, 268

High Blood Pressure - Hawthorn, 229; Garlic, 207; Valerian, 409

Hormonal Acne - Chaste Tree, 145; Spearmint, 379

Hormonal Balance - Ashwagandha, 98; Angelica, 92;
  Chaste Tree, 145; Dong Quai, 178; Wild Yam, 423; Chaste Tree, 145

Hypertensive (anti) - Garlic, 207; Hawthorn, 229

Hyperthyroidism Management - Lemon Balm, 258

Hypothalamus Regulation - Ashwagandha, 98; Skullcap, 367

Hypothyroidism Support - Ashwagandha, 98

Immune System Support - Astragalus, 101; Echinacea, 182;
  Elderberry, 186

Indigestion - Fennel, 196; Peppermint, 322

Infection Prevention - Astragalus, 101; Echinacea, 182; Garlic, 207

Infections - Goldenseal, 222; Echinacea, 182

Inflammation (arthritis, joint pain) - Turmeric, 402; Ginger, 211

Inflammation - (joints/skin) - Chamomile, 142; Turmeric, 402

Insect Bites - Plantain, 330; Lavender, 254; Calendula, 123

Insomnia - Valerian, 409; Chamomile, 142

Insulin Release Stimulation - Fenugreek, 200

Insulin Sensitivity (response) - Cinnamon, 159; Fenugreek, 200

Intestines - Slippery Elm, 370; Marshmallow Root, 282

Joint Pain - Turmeric, 402; Ginger, 211

Joint Support - Turmeric, 402; Ginger, 211; Nettle, 304

Kidney Health - Dandelion, 174; Burdock, 120; Parsley, 316;
  Nettle, 304

Kidney Stone Prevention - Horsetail, 244; Lemon Balm, 258;
  Dandelion, 174

Libido Enhancement - Damiana, 170; Ashwagandha, 98

Ligament Strength - Horsetail, 244; Nettle, 304

Liver Health - Milk Thistle, 288; Dandelion, 174; Burdock, 120

Lungs - Anise, 95; Echinacea, 182; Elecampane, 189; Fennel, 196; Fenugreek, 200; Ginger, 211; Horehound, 240; Hyssop, 247; Licorice, 268; Mullein, 298; Thyme, 398

Lymph Flow - Echinacea, 182; Red Clover, 341

Lymph Node Health - Echinacea, 182

Lymphatic Cancer Support - Turmeric, 402; Echinacea, 182

Lymphatic Circulation Improvement - Calendula, 123; Red Clover, 341

Lymphatic Cleansing - Nettle, 304; Dandelion, 174; Burdock, 120

Lymphatic Congestion - Red Clover, 341

Lymphatic Drainage - Calendula, 123; Mullein, 298

Lymphatic Filtration Improvement - Red Clover, 341; Echinacea, 182

Lymphatic Fluid Balance - Dandelion, 174; Nettle, 304

Lymphatic System Detox - Burdock, 120; Red Clover, 341

Lymphatic Tissue Repair - Calendula, 123; Yarrow, 429

Lymphoma Care - Astragalus, 101; Echinacea, 182; Turmeric, 402

Memory Enhancement - Ginkgo Biloba, 214; Rosemary, 351

Menopause Support - Sage, 358; Red Clover, 341; Dong Quai, 178

Menopause Symptoms - Red Clover, 341; Dong Quai, 178

Menstrual Cycle Regulation - Chaste Tree, 145; Dong Quai, 178; Angelica, 92

Menstrual Relief - Ginger, 211; Peppermint, 322; Chamomile, 142; Yarrow, 429

Mental Clarity - Ginkgo Biloba, 214; Rosemary, 351

Mental Fatigue - Rhodiola Rosea, 344

Metabolism Boost - Ginseng, 218

Migraines - Feverfew, 204; Peppermint, 322

Mood Swings - St. John's Wort, 389; Ashwagandha, 98

Muscle Relaxation - Lavender, 254; Chamomile, 142; Valerian, 409

Nasal Passages - Peppermint, 322; Yarrow, 429

Nausea - Ginger, 211; Peppermint, 322

Nerve Calming - Lemon Balm, 258; Chamomile, 142; Valerian, 409

Nerve Pain - St. John's Wort, 389; Skullcap, 367

Nerve Regeneration - St. John's Wort, 389; Gotu Kola, 226

Nerve Support - St. John's Wort, 389; Skullcap, 367

Nervous System Health - Skullcap, 367; Ashwagandha, 98

Nervousness - Catnip, 134; Passionflower, 319

Neuralgia - St. John's Wort, 389; Chamomile, 142

Neurological Health - Ginkgo Biloba, 214; Gotu Kola, 226

Neuropathy Health - St. John's Wort, 389; Skullcap, 367

Neuroprotection - Ashwagandha, 98; Ginkgo Biloba, 214

Nose/Nasal Passages - Peppermint, 322; Yarrow, 429

Oil Regulation (Skin) - Witch Hazel, 426; Lavender, 254; Rosemary, 351

Osteoporosis Prevention - Red Clover, 341; Horsetail, 244; Nettle, 304

Ovaries Support - Chaste Tree, 145; Dong Quai, 178; Angelica, 92

Pain Relief - Turmeric, 402

Pancreas Function - Fenugreek, 200

Pathogen Defense - Echinacea, 182; Garlic, 207

PH balance - Lemon Balm, 258

Pineal Gland Function - Lavender, 254

Pituitary Function - Ashwagandha, 98

PMS Relief - Chaste Tree, 145; Dong Quai, 178; Lemon Balm, 258

Pore Minimizing - Witch Hazel, 426; Lavender, 254; Thyme, 398

Postpartum Recovery - Motherwort, 295; Raspberry Leaf, 338; Nettle, 304

Pregnancy Support - Raspberry Leaf, 338; Nettle, 304; Ginger, 211

Progesterone Production - Chaste Tree, 145; Wild Yam, 423

Prostate Health - Nettle, 304

Psoriasis Relief - Neem, 301; Turmeric, 402; Chamomile, 142

Rash Treatment - Chamomile, 142; Calendula, 123; Lavender, 254

Respiratory Health - Echinacea, 182; Mullein, 298

Respiratory Infections - Echinacea, 182; Elderberry, 186; Thyme, 398

Respiratory Mucosa - Marshmallow Root, 282; Slippery Elm, 370

Respiratory Relaxant - Chamomile, 142; Lavender, 254; Lemon Balm, 258

Respiratory Strength - Astragalus, 101

Rheumatism Treatment - Nettle, 304; Burdock, 120

Scar Reduction - Lavender, 254; Rosemary, 351; Calendula, 123

Sinus infections - Echinacea, 182; Goldenseal, 222; Elderberry, 186

Sinus Health - Elderberry, 186; Peppermint, 322; Yarrow, 429

Skin Brightening - Lemon; Licorice, 268; Chamomile, 142

Skin Detox - Burdock, 120; Dandelion, 174; Milk Thistle, 288

Skin Elasticity - Gotu Kola, 226; Horsetail, 244; Aloe Vera, 89

Skin Healing - Aloe Vera, 89; Calendula, 123; Comfrey

Skin Health - Aloe Vera, 89; Calendula, 123; Chamomile, 142

Skin Hydration - Aloe Vera, 89; Lavender, 254; Calendula, 123

Skin Infections - Aloe Vera, 89; Calendula, 123; Chamomile, 142; Echinacea, 182; Garlic, 207; Goldenseal, 222; Goldenseal, 222; Lavender, 254; Oregano, 312; Thyme, 398

Skin Inflammation Reduction - Turmeric, 402; Chamomile, 142; Lavender, 254

Skin Nourishment - Lavender, 254; Chamomile, 142

Skin Redness Reduction - Aloe Vera, 89; Chamomile, 142

Skin Repair - Lavender, 254; Plantain, 330; Yarrow, 429

Skin Texture - Lavender, 254; Rosemary, 351; Chamomile, 142

Sleep Disorders - Valerian, 409; Lemon Balm, 258

Sleep Regulation - Valerian, 409; Passionflower, 319; Lemon Balm, 258

Spasm Relief - Valerian, 409; Chamomile, 142; Peppermint, 322

Sperm Health - Ashwagandha, 98; Ginseng, 218

Spleen Support - Astragalus, 101; Dandelion, 174; Milk Thistle, 288

Stomach Health - Aloe Vera, 89; Angelica, 92; Basil, 104

Stomach Lining - Aloe Vera, 89; Slippery Elm, 370

Strength Support - Ashwagandha, 98; Astragalus, 101

Stress Relief - Ashwagandha, 98; Holy Basil, 232; Lemon Balm, 258

Stroke - Ginkgo Biloba, 214; Hawthorn, 229; Turmeric, 402

Sun Protection - Lavender, 254; Aloe Vera, 89

Swelling Reduction (lymphatic) - Witch Hazel, 426; Yarrow, 429

Tension Relief - Lavender, 254; Chamomile, 142; Lemon Balm, 258; Valerian, 409

Testicular Function - Ashwagandha, 98

Testosterone Boost - Tribulus; Fenugreek, 200; Ashwagandha, 98

Throat - Chamomile, 142; Licorice, 268; Marshmallow Root, 282; Sage, 358; Slippery Elm, 370

Thyroid Antibody Reduction - Ashwagandha, 98

Thyroid Hormone Synthesis - Ashwagandha, 98

Thyroid Support - Ashwagandha, 98; Nettle, 304

Tiredness - Ginseng, 218; Ashwagandha, 98; Rhodiola Rosea, 344

Toothache, Gum Health - Clove, 163; Chamomile, 142; Echinacea, 182

Ulcers - Aloe Vera, 89

Urinary Antiseptic - Echinacea, 182

Uterine Health - Raspberry Leaf, 338; Motherwort, 295; Red Clover, 341

Uterine Toning - Raspberry Leaf, 338; Nettle, 304; Motherwort, 295

UTI Relief - Dandelion, 174; Horsetail, 244; Echinacea, 182

Vaginal Health - Goldenseal, 222; Aloe Vera, 89

Veins, Varicose - Witch Hazel, 426; Yarrow, 429

Viral Infections - Lemon Balm, 258; Echinacea, 182; Oregano, 312

Wound Healing - Calendula, 123; Yarrow, 429; Aloe Vera, 89

Contents

Part III
Herbal Remedies for Health and Wellness

≫ **Understanding Herbal Properties** - How herbs interact with your different body systems.

→ Teas and Infusions

→ Tinctures

→ Salves - Topical Applications (creams/ointments/poultices)

→ Compresses

→ Aromatherapy & Essential Oils

→ Herbal Baths

→ Steam Inhalation

→ Decoctions

→ Syrups

→ Gargles and Mouthwashes

→ Powders

→ Juices

Advice on determining the right dosage for different herbs and the safest methods for administering them.

≫ **Safety and Precautions** - Information on potential side effects, interactions with medications, and when to avoid certain herbs.

≫ **Herbal Combination Formulas** - Step-by-Step Instructions on how to combine different herbs to create effective herbal remedies.

≫ **Customizing Remedies** - Tailoring herbal treatments to individual needs, including considerations for age, constitution, and specific health conditions.

- ≫ **Labeling and Documentation** - Keeping detailed records of herbal remedies prepared, including ingredients, dates, and usage instructions.
- ≫ **Storage and Preservation** - Best practices for storing herbs to maintain their potency, including drying, freezing, and using appropriate containers.
- ≫ **Purchasing Herbs from Outside Sources** - Emphasizing the importance of ethical sourcing and sustainable practices in herbalism.

- ≫ **Pairing Herbs with Foods for Flavor and Health**
- ≫ **Creative Uses of Herbs in Beverages**
- ≫ **Creating Seasonings, Spices and Condiments**

- ≫ **Herbs for Stress, Anxiety, and Sleep Disorders**
  Natural solutions to manage stress, reduce anxiety, and improve sleep, enhancing overall well-being and mental health.
- ≫ **Incorporating Therapeutic Gardening Practices into Daily Life**

Part IV
Urban/City Herbal Gardening

- → Balconies
- → Windowsills
- → Indoor Gardens
- → Artificial Indoor Lighting

Part V
100 BEST Herbs to Grow

➜ Overwintering
➜ Propagation
➜ Harvesting
➜ Climate Considerations

≫ **How to Use 100:**
☐ Teas and Infusions
☐ Tinctures
☐ Salves - Topical Applications
(creams/ointments/poultices)
☐ Compresses
☐ Aromatherapy & Essential Oils
☐ Baths
☐ Steam Inhalation
☐ Decoctions
☐ Syrups
☐ Gargles and Mouthwashes
☐ Powders
☐ Juices
☐ Culinary Uses

≫ **Ease to Grow Scale** (Each Plant Rated)
Low Maintenance: 1-3
Medium Maintenance: 4-6
High Maintenance: 7-9
Expert Level: 10

Introduction

Isn't it incredible that the medicines and remedies science has developed to heal us all originate from the earth? Think about it: two thousand years ago, we couldn't just plant and harvest aspirin, penicillin, or the myriad of chemicals and compounds we have today. From over-the-counter drugs to doctor's prescriptions, where do they all come from? They've always been right here, with an astonishing variety of herbs and natural remedies growing all around us.

But here's the thing—there are thousands of them! How do we figure out which herbs are best for specific health issues? How can we be sure that what we're growing will actually work as medicine? And how should we harvest and prepare these plants and herbs to make them part of our daily health routine? This book will uncover these mysteries for you, looking deep into each of our body's physiological systems and even further into our individual organs and components these herbs benefit.

But we can't stop there; that's just half the battle. Do you know how to start growing plants and herbs, even in limited spaces? Together we'll walk through the entire process step-by-step; from choosing the right herb for your needs to understanding the perfect soil mix, lighting, feeding, watering and more. Whether you'll be starting with seeds or plants, we'll also cover: pruning and maintenance, what pests and diseases to watch out for, and how to propagate (expand) your plants.

Next, you'll find specific information on harvesting, preparing, and using each herb—whether it's the flowers, stems, leaves, roots, or seeds—whenever beneficial.

Learn which herbs are best for creating: herbal teas, tinctures, salves, aromatherapy & essential oils, herbal baths, decoctions, syrups and juices... PLUS plants that can be used in food preparation, and how each is most commonly consumed. Each of the 100 plants will also be rated on a unique 'ease-to-grow' scale from 1 to 10, so you can match your skill level (or the time you have available) to help each plant thrive.

As we begin to implement herbal medicine and gardening, remember that the ability to heal and nurture is within your reach, right in our own gardens and homes. Let's start this journey together, learning and growing with each plant we cultivate, and equipping ourselves with the knowledge to lead healthier lives naturally.

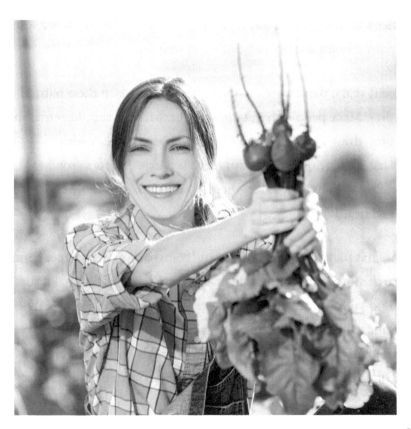

Part I
Introduction to Herbal Medicine

1. The Rise of Herbal Medicine

Herbal medicine is not just a trend; it's a tradition that has stood the test of time. Its journey from ancient practices to modern-day popularity is a fascinating story of human connection with nature and the wisdom passed down through generations.

Long before pharmacies and prescriptions, our ancestors found healing in the natural world, using plants to treat various ailments. This deep-rooted knowledge formed the basis of herbal medicine, a practice that has evolved but remains grounded in the understanding that nature holds the key to health and wellness.

In recent years, there's been a noticeable shift back to these natural remedies. More people are reaching for herbal teas, supplements, and tinctures, drawn by the appeal of treating health issues with plant-based solutions. This resurgence is partly due to a growing skepticism of conventional medicine and a desire for more control over personal health care.

Science has played a crucial role in the comeback of herbal medicine. Research studies are continually backing up what traditional healers have known for centuries: plants have powerful healing properties. Scientific validation has helped bridge the gap between ancient wisdom and modern skepticism, giving herbal medicine a renewed sense of credibility and acceptance in the health community.

Herbal medicine's applications are as diverse as the plants themselves. From soothing anxiety and promoting sleep with chamomile to boosting the immune system with echinacea, the range of uses is vast. This versatility makes herbal medicine a valuable tool in both preventive health and the treatment of chronic conditions.

Culturally, the use of herbal remedies is a reflection of a broader interest in sustainable living and wellness. Across the globe, different cultures have their unique herbal traditions, which are now being shared and appreciated on a wider scale. This cultural exchange enriches the practice of herbal medicine, bringing a variety of perspectives and remedies to the table.

The holistic approach of herbal medicine is another factor in its rising popularity. Unlike conventional treatments that often focus on symptoms, herbalism looks at the entire person, considering physical, mental, and emotional health. This comprehensive view aligns with the growing interest in wellness and the recognition that health is multidimensional.

However, the path of herbal medicine is not without challenges. Regulation, quality control, and the potential for misinformation are significant hurdles. As the demand for herbal products increases, ensuring they are safe, effective, and sustainably sourced becomes increasingly important.

There's also the challenge of integrating herbal medicine into mainstream health care. While some progress has been made, there's still a long way to go in bridging traditional and modern practices, ensuring that people have access to the best of both worlds.

Despite these challenges, the opportunities for herbal medicine are vast. As research continues and public interest grows, there's potential for greater acceptance and integration of herbal remedies in health care systems. This could lead to more personalized, natural, and holistic treatment options, benefiting individuals and communities alike.

In short, the growing interest in herbal medicine shows our desire for natural and sustainable health care. From its historical beginnings to its current popularity, supported by science and cultural traditions, herbal medicine is a dynamic and evolving field. It has the potential to change how we think about and manage our health. As we face new challenges and seize opportunities, the future of herbal medicine looks bright, offering a health path that's in tune with nature and the wisdom of past generations.

2. Understanding Herbal Medicine

Basics of Herbalism and its Benefits:

Herbalism is like tapping into nature's own medicine cabinet, where each plant holds a key to better health and well-being. It's an ancient practice that humans have relied on for thousands of years, and today, it's making a huge comeback as more people seek natural alternatives to conventional medicine.

So, what's the big deal with herbalism? Well, for starters, it's all about using plants to promote health, prevent illness, and treat various conditions. Unlike modern drugs that often target specific symptoms, herbs work on a holistic level, supporting the body's natural healing processes.

Herbs for Health

- **Natural and Gentle:** Herbs offer a softer, more natural way to support health without the harsh side effects often associated with prescription drugs.
- **Holistic Healing:** Herbalism looks at the whole person, not just the disease, promoting overall well-being.
- **Preventive Care:** Regular use of certain herbs can strengthen the immune system and prevent illnesses.

Economic and Accessible

- **Cost-Effective:** Growing your own herbs can save money on healthcare costs and store-bought remedies.
- **Easy to Access:** Many medicinal herbs are easy to grow at home, making them readily available when needed.

Sustainable and Eco-Friendly

- **Environmentally Friendly:** Using locally grown herbs reduces the environmental impact associated with transporting and manufacturing pharmaceuticals.
- **Promotes Biodiversity:** Cultivating a variety of herbs can support local plant life and animal life.

Personal Empowerment

- **Self-Sufficiency:** Learning to use herbs for health care fosters independence from the conventional medical system.
- **Knowledge and Skills:** Gaining knowledge about herbal remedies empowers individuals to make informed health decisions.

Cultural and Historical Significance

- **Cultural Heritage:** Herbalism is part of many cultural traditions and reconnects individuals with their ancestral roots.
- **Historical Wisdom:** Utilizing herbs for healing draws on centuries of accumulated knowledge and experience.

But how exactly do herbs work their magic? They're packed with a variety of compounds that have specific effects on the body. Some herbs have anti-inflammatory properties, others are antiviral or antibacterial, and some can soothe the nervous system or aid digestion. The key is knowing which herb to use for what purpose.

Herbalism isn't just about treating illness, though. It's also a proactive approach to maintaining health. Incorporating herbs into daily life, through teas, cooking, or supplements, can boost overall vitality and prevent health issues before they start.

Now, you might be thinking, "This all sounds great, but is it really for me?" Absolutely! Herbalism is for everyone. Whether you're dealing with chronic health issues, looking to boost your immune system, or simply interested in living a more natural lifestyle, there's a place for herbs in your life.

Getting started with herbalism can be as simple as brewing a cup of chamomile tea to relax before bed or using aloe vera for skin irritation. As you become more comfortable, you might venture into making your own herbal tinctures, salves, or syrups.

One of the best things about herbalism is the sense of community it fosters. There are countless resources available, from books and websites to workshops and herb walks, allowing you to learn from experienced herbalists and connect with others who share your interest.

In summary, herbalism offers a world of benefits, from improving health and saving money to supporting the environment and connecting with cultural traditions. It enables people to take control of their health care in a natural, holistic way. So, whether you're a seasoned herbal enthusiast or just starting, there's never been a better time to explore the wonderful world of herbalism.

People, Plants, & Health, all Connected

The link between us, plants, and our health is really something special. It's not just about fixing a health problem here and there; it's about the whole picture of feeling good, both in mind and body. This idea isn't new—it's been around since the days when traditional medicine first turned to plants for healing.

Having plants around, whether we're using them as herbal remedies or just enjoying a green space, can seriously lift our spirits and clear our minds. And it's not just about feeling better; it's about doing right by the planet too. Growing herbs in a way that's good for the earth helps make sure we can keep using these green goodies without running out.

Learning about herbs isn't just smart; it's invigorating. It means we get to take charge of our health, understanding what works for us and why. And let's not forget about food. Bringing more plants into our meals is a tasty way to boost our health big time.

When we come together as a community to share our love for herbal goodness, it's even better. It's like tapping into a well of knowledge and tradition, keeping alive the age-old wisdom of using plants to feel better.

In a nutshell, our bond with plants is all about living well, respecting nature, and learning from each other. It's amazing how these leafy friends of ours can play such a big part in our health and happiness.

Part II
Getting Started with Your Herbal Garden

3. Planning Your Herbal Garden

Assessing Your Space and Resources:

Starting your herbal garden is like setting up a new home for your plant friends, and just like any good home, it needs the right space and resources. Before you get started planting, it's crucial to take a good look at what you've got to work with. This isn't just about having a patch of dirt; it's about creating the perfect environment for your herbs to flourish.

First up, let's talk about space. Not everyone has a sprawling garden, and that's okay! Herbs are pretty accommodating and can thrive in various settings. Whether you have a backyard, a small balcony, or just a windowsill, there's a way to make it work. The key is understanding the space you have and how you can best utilize it. For instance:

- **Backyard Gardens:** Offer plenty of room for a variety of herbs. You can design larger beds and even create different zones for various types of plants.
- **Balconies and Patios:** Ideal for container gardening. Pots and planters can house a surprising number of herbs, making efficient use of limited outdoor space.
- **Indoor and Windowsill Gardens:** Perfect for herbs that don't need too much sunlight or can thrive indoors, like mint or chives.

Next is sunlight. Herbs love the sun, but each type has its own preference for how much light it needs. Some, like basil and rosemary, are sun worshippers and crave lots of direct light. Others, such as parsley and cilantro, can handle shadier spots. Assessing the sunlight your space receives will guide you in choosing the right herbs for your garden. Here's what to consider:

- **Direct Sunlight Areas:** Best for herbs that need 6-8 hours of sunlight daily.
- **Partial Shade Areas:** Suitable for herbs that prefer less intense sun exposure.
- **Indoor Light:** If natural light is limited, artificial grow lights can supplement the light needed for healthy growth.

Water is another crucial element. All plants of course need water, but the amount and frequency depend on the herb type and your local climate. Some herbs are drought-tolerant, like lavender and thyme, while others, such as basil, need consistent moisture. Here are some water-related points to ponder:

- **Natural Rainfall:** Consider how much rain your area typically gets and if additional watering will be necessary.
- **Irrigation and Watering Systems:** In drier climates or for container gardens, setting up a reliable watering system can save time and ensure your plants get the hydration they need.

Soil quality can make or break your garden. Herbs generally prefer well-draining soil with a neutral to slightly acidic pH. However, some might need specific soil types or additions to thrive. Assessing your soil can involve:

- **Soil Testing:** Check the pH level and nutrient content to see if you need to adjust it with compounds or choose plants suited to the existing conditions.

- **Container Gardening:** If your natural soil isn't ideal or you're gardening in pots, using a high-quality potting mix can provide your herbs with the right environment to grow.

Lastly, consider your own resources and time. Gardening is a commitment, and you want to make sure it fits into your lifestyle. Think about:

- **Time Availability:** How much time can you realistically dedicate to maintaining your garden? Choose herbs that fit your schedule, whether they need daily attention or can thrive with less frequent care.
- **Budget:** Factor in the cost of seeds, soil, pots, tools, and other gardening supplies. Starting small and expanding as you go can be a budget-friendly approach.

By assessing your space and resources, you can create a thriving herbal garden that suits your environment and lifestyle. It's all about making informed choices and planning ahead to ensure your herbal adventure is successful and enjoyable.

Selecting the right herbs for your needs and environment:

Choosing the right herbs to grow at home is like picking new friends who will support and nourish you. It's all about finding those that fit well with your lifestyle, health needs, and the space you have available. Just as you consider compatibility in relationships, you should think about how the herbs you choose will interact with your life and the environment you can provide for them.

Firstly, consider what you need from your herbal buddies. Are you looking for herbs to help you relax, like lavender or chamomile? Or do you need something to boost your immune system, such as echinacea or elderberry? Identifying your health priorities will guide you in selecting herbs that serve your specific needs.

Next, think about the space you have. Not all herbs require a garden; many thrive in pots on windowsills or balconies. Mint, basil, and cilantro, for example, are great for small spaces and can easily be grown indoors. If you have a yard or garden, you might opt for larger plants like lemon balm or rosemary, which can spread out and even become perennial fixtures in your landscape.

Your local climate is another crucial factor. Some herbs are hearty and can handle different weather conditions, while others might need a more controlled environment. Researching the herbs that naturally thrive in your area can lead to more successful gardening. For instance, if you live in a cooler climate, you might lean towards plants like peppermint or chives, which are more cold-tolerant.

In essence, choosing the right herbs involves aligning your health goals with the practicalities of your living situation and local climate. By doing so, you create a personalized herbal garden that not only grows well but also brings the specific health benefits you're seeking.

4. Essential Tools and Techniques

Gardening Tools and Their Uses:

Gardening requires the right tools to get the job done efficiently and effectively. Here's a straightforward look at some essential gardening tools and what they're used for:

- **Shovels and Spades:** Essential for digging, turning the soil, and planting. They are the foundational tools for creating and preparing garden beds.
- **Garden Fork:** Ideal for loosening and aerating the soil, as well as integrating compost or other organic matter to enrich the soil quality.
- **Hoe:** A vital tool for weed control and soil aeration. It's used to maintain clear soil surfaces and manage weed growth without using chemicals.
- **Hand Trowel:** Handy for more precise work like planting smaller plants, bulbs, or doing detailed soil work in tighter spaces.
- **Pruning Shears:** Necessary for trimming and shaping plants, removing dead or overgrown branches, and maintaining the health and aesthetics of your garden.
- **Watering Can or Hose:** Ensures your plants receive the necessary hydration. The choice between a can or hose depends on the size of your garden and the specific watering needs of your plants.

Having these tools at your disposal will help you manage your garden more effectively, keeping it healthy and vibrant. Whether you're establishing a new garden or maintaining an existing one, these tools are fundamental to achieving gardening success.

Basic Gardening Techniques Tailored to Medicinal Plants

Gardening isn't just about throwing seeds in the ground and hoping for the best, especially when it comes to medicinal plants. These special plants need a bit more care to make sure they provide the health benefits we're looking for. Later on in the individual herb section, we'll provide more specific growing instructions pertinent to each specific plant.

For now, let's break down some general gardening techniques that will help your medicinal plants thrive.

- **Soil Prep:** Medicinal plants often need well-draining soil rich in organic matter. Before planting, work in compost or aged manure to boost nutrients. This gives your plants a strong start.
- **Proper Spacing:** Giving plants enough room is crucial. Crowded plants can struggle to get enough light and air circulation, which can lead to disease. Check the specific spacing needs for each individual herb (listed later in this book) to ensure they have room to grow strong and healthy.
- **Watering Wisely:** Overwatering can be just as harmful as under-watering. Most medicinal herbs prefer soil that's moist but not soggy. Water deeply but infrequently to encourage strong root development.

- **Sunlight:** Most herbs love the sun, requiring around 6 to 8 hours of direct light daily. Position your garden or containers where they can bask in plenty of natural light. If you're growing indoors, a sunny windowsill or artificial grow lights can do the trick (more info on specific lighting needs later with each plant).
- **Pruning and Harvesting:** Regular pruning helps plants bush out and produce more of the good stuff—leaves, flowers, or roots that we use for remedies. Learn the best times to harvest each plant, as the timing can affect the potency of its medicinal properties.
- **Pest Management:** Keeping an eye out for pests and dealing with them early is key. Often, a blast of water from a hose or natural remedies like neem oil can manage pests without resorting to harsh chemicals.

By honing in on these simple techniques, you're laying down a solid base for your medicinal garden. But it's not just about planting herbs; think of it as cultivating your very own backyard pharmacy. With some basic knowledge and a bit of tender care, your garden will become more than just plants—it'll be a go-to spot for health and healing, offering natural remedies that support a well-rounded approach to wellness.

5. From Planting to Harvesting

Planting, Growing, and Harvesting Herbs

Growing herbs is like embarking on a green adventure where you get to play with dirt and end up with a bounty of fragrant and healing plants. Let's walk through a little on planting, growing, and harvesting your herbal treasures.

Planning Your Herb Garden

Before you start, think about what herbs you want to grow. Consider your health needs, culinary preferences, and the space you have. Do you want herbs for soothing teas, like chamomile and mint, or culinary stars like basil and thyme? Once you've picked your favorites, it's time to get your hands dirty.

Planting Your Herbs

You can start herbs from seeds or buy young plants (or starts) from a nursery. If starting from seeds:

- **Sowing Seeds:** Plant them in small pots or trays with seed-starting mix. Keep the soil moist but not waterlogged, and place them in a warm, bright spot until they germinate.
- **Transplanting:** Once seedlings are big enough to handle and the danger of frost has passed, transplant them to your garden or larger containers, spacing them as recommended.

For Nursery Plants

- **Acclimatizing:** Let your plants get used to outdoor conditions by placing them outside for a few hours each day for a week before planting.
- **Planting Out:** Dig a hole big enough for the root ball, place the plant in, fill in with soil, and water well.

Caring for Your Herb Garden

Herbs are relatively low-maintenance, but they still need some TLC to flourish. More specifics for each plant in Chapter 12.

- **Watering:** Water your herbs when the soil feels dry an inch below the surface. Early morning is the best time to water, giving plants plenty of moisture before the heat of the day.
- **Feeding:** Use a balanced, organic fertilizer sparingly. Herbs don't need much to grow, and too much can reduce their flavor and medicinal properties.
- **Mulching:** A layer of mulch helps retain moisture, suppress weeds, and keep the soil temperature stable.

Dealing with Pests and Problems

Keep an eye out for any signs of pests or disease. Natural remedies, like neem oil or insecticidal soap, can handle most common garden pests. Healthy, well-cared-for plants are less likely to succumb to diseases.

Pruning and Maintenance

Regular pruning not only keeps your plants tidy but also encourages more growth.

- **Pinching Back:** Pinch off the tips of your herbs to encourage bushier growth. This is especially good for basil, mint, and cilantro.
- **Harvesting Leaves:** Always leave enough leaves on the plant to ensure it can continue to photosynthesize and grow.

Harvesting Your Herbs

- **Optimal Harvest Time:** Aim for the early morning hours, after the dew has settled but before the full intensity of the sun. This is when the herbs' essential oils, responsible for flavor and aroma, are at their peak concentration. The cooler morning temperature helps preserve these oils, ensuring you capture the herbs' full sensory and therapeutic benefits.
- **Leaf Harvesting:** Gather leaves before the herb plants flower, as this is when the leaves contain the highest levels of active compounds and flavors. The stage just before flowering is crucial because the plant's energy is focused on leaf growth, resulting in richer, more potent leaves.
- **Flower Harvesting:** Pick the flowers when they are fully bloomed but before they begin to fade or wilt. This timing ensures you get the flowers at their most vibrant, when they are packed with essential oils and active ingredients. The flowers should be plump, colorful, and fragrant, indicating they are at their freshest and most beneficial.
- **Seed Harvesting:** Collect seeds when they have matured and the seed heads have dried out, usually turning a brownish

color. Mature seeds have had time to develop fully, encapsulating the plant's properties effectively. Waiting for the seed heads to dry on the plant allows the seeds to achieve their full medicinal and culinary potential, ensuring you harvest them at the right time for maximum potency.

Storing Your Harvest
(Much more on storage in the next chapter)

You can use fresh herbs straight from the garden, but if you have a surplus, consider drying or freezing them for later use.

- **Drying:** Hang bunches of herbs upside down in a warm, dry place away from direct sunlight. Once dry, strip the leaves or flowers from the stems and store in airtight containers.
- **Freezing:** Chop fresh herbs and freeze them in ice cube trays with water or oil, perfect for throwing into soups or stews.

Growing herbs is a rewarding experience, offering not just the satisfaction of gardening but also the joy of harvesting your own natural remedies and culinary enhancers. With a bit of planning and care, your garden can become a verdant source of health and flavor, ready to enrich your life and your meals.

Seasonal Care and Maintenance Tips

Taking care of medicinal herbs isn't just a spring or summer task; it's a year-round commitment. Each season brings its own set of challenges and opportunities for your herb garden, so let's look at how you can keep your green buddies happy and healthy throughout the year.

When the weather shifts, so should your watering routine. During hot summer days, your herbs might need more frequent watering to combat the heat, while in cooler months, they'll require less. It's all about observing the weather and adjusting your watering schedule accordingly to prevent over or under-watering.

*Mulching is like giving your herbs a cozy blanket. It helps regulate soil temperature, keeping roots cool in summer and warm in winter. Plus, it retains moisture, so you won't have to water as often, and it keeps those annoying weeds at bay.

***Mulching refers to the act of covering soil with materials like organic matter or plastic to improve plant growth and soil health.**

Fertilizing isn't a one-time event; it should match your herbs' growth stages. Sprinkle some organic fertilizer or compost during the growing season to give them a nutrient boost, helping them grow lush and hearty.

The timing of planting and harvesting can also change with the seasons. Some herbs prefer the cool start of spring, while others thrive in the summer heat. And when it comes to harvesting, pay attention to weather cues. Sometimes, an unexpected frost or a sudden heatwave can mean you need to harvest sooner than planned.

Don't forget about the sun! Herbs love sunlight, but too much can be harsh, especially in the peak of summer. Providing some shade can prevent them from getting scorched. Conversely, in cooler months, make sure they get enough light to keep growing.

Aerating the soil and rotating your crops are also key. Compacted soil can hinder root growth, so give it a little fluff-up now and then. And by rotating where you plant your herbs, you help keep the soil healthy and reduce the risk of disease and pest buildup.

By keeping these seasonal care tips in mind, you can ensure your medicinal herb garden remains vibrant and productive all year round, providing you with fresh, healing plants for your needs.

Part III
Herbal Remedies for Health and Wellness

6. Creating Your Herbal Pharmacy

Understanding Herbal Properties:

Herbs are nature's way of supporting our health and well-being, each packed with unique properties that can help us feel better. Think of them as friends with special skills; some might soothe an upset stomach, while others can calm a busy mind or heal a skin irritation.

Active Ingredients

Herbs are packed with natural compounds that have various effects on our body. Take ginger, for example, which contains gingerol. This compound is a powerhouse for aiding digestion and battling nausea. Similarly, turmeric's curcumin is known for its anti-inflammatory and antioxidant properties. Understanding these active ingredients helps in selecting the right herb for the right ailment, ensuring effective and targeted healing.

Targeted Support

Herbs have affinities for specific body systems, making them incredibly useful for targeted healing. Echinacea, for example, is famous for stimulating the immune system, making it a go-to herb during cold and flu season. On the other hand, hawthorn is often used for its cardiovascular benefits, helping to regulate blood pressure and support heart health. By knowing which herb affects which body system, you can create a personalized herbal regimen that addresses specific health concerns.

Synergy Effect

The power of herbs is magnified when they are used in combination. This "synergy" allows the herbs to work together, enhancing their individual effects. For instance, combining chamomile and lavender can create a potent blend for relaxation and stress relief, more effective than using each herb alone. This synergistic approach in herbal medicine not only maximizes the therapeutic benefits but also can reduce the needed dosage of each herb, minimizing potential side effects.

Preparation Matters

The way herbs are prepared can greatly influence their healing properties. Tea, for instance, offers a mild and accessible form of the herb's benefits, ideal for daily maintenance of health. Tinctures, being more concentrated, provide a stronger dose and can be more effective for acute conditions. Capsules offer convenience and dosage accuracy. Each preparation method has its place, and understanding this can help in choosing the most suitable form for one's health needs.

Personalization

Herbal medicine is not one-size-fits-all. What works wonderfully for one person might be less effective or unsuitable for another. Personal factors like age, health condition, and even genetics play a role in how an individual responds to herbs. It's important to experiment carefully and observe your body's reactions, possibly under the guidance of a healthcare professional, to tailor herbal treatment to your specific needs and circumstances. This personalization is key to achieving the best therapeutic outcomes with herbal medicine.

Preparation and Use Techniques:

Teas and Infusions

How to Make: Start by selecting your preferred herb, either fresh or dried, noting the difference in potency (fresh herbs are less concentrated than dried). Use one tablespoon of fresh herbs or one teaspoon of dried herbs per cup of water. Boil the water and pour it over the herbs in a teapot or jar, ensuring they are fully submerged. Cover the container to prevent the escape of steam and volatile oils, which contain the therapeutic properties of the herbs. Allow the herbs to steep for at least 5 to 15 minutes; for a stronger infusion, you can leave them for up to 30 minutes. This extended steeping time allows more of the active compounds to be extracted into the water.

How to Use: Once steeped, strain the mixture to remove the solid herb parts. The resulting liquid can be consumed as a tea, either hot or chilled, depending on personal preference. For therapeutic use, drinking herbal tea can support various body functions, from digestion to stress relief. The tea can also be applied externally as a wash for skin irritations, used as a gargle for soothing throat infections, or employed as an eye compress for tired or inflamed eyes, providing a versatile remedy from a single preparation.

Tinctures

How to Make: Begin by finely chopping or grinding the chosen herbs to maximize the surface area exposed to the solvent, which enhances the extraction of active ingredients. Place the prepared herbs in a clean glass jar, filling it about two-thirds full. Pour a suitable solvent, such as alcohol (vodka or brandy) or apple cider vinegar, over the herbs until they are completely submerged. This solvent acts as a preservative and extraction agent, pulling the active compounds out of the plant material. Seal the jar tightly and label it with the herb name, type of solvent, and date. Store the jar in a cool, dark place to protect it from light and heat, which can degrade the tincture's quality. Shake the jar daily to agitate the mixture and facilitate the extraction process. Allow the tincture to macerate for about 4 to 6 weeks, which gives enough time for the solvent to dissolve the plant's active compounds.

How to Use: After the maceration (soaking) period, strain the liquid through a fine mesh sieve or cheesecloth to separate the herb particles from the liquid tincture. Transfer the strained tincture to a clean, dark glass bottle for storage. Administer the tincture using a dropper, placing drops directly under the tongue for rapid absorption into the bloodstream, which bypasses the digestive system and allows for quicker therapeutic effects. Tinctures can also be diluted in water or tea if the taste is too strong or for ease of consumption. The concentrated nature of tinctures makes them a potent form of herbal medicine, effective for a wide range of health conditions, from digestive issues to stress and anxiety relief.

Topical Applications

(Creams and Ointments)

How to Make: The process involves gently heating a chosen herb in a carrier oil, such as coconut, almond, or olive oil, to extract the active constituents of the herb into the oil. This is done over low heat for several hours, ensuring that the oil does not overheat, which could degrade the therapeutic properties of the herbs. After the herbs have infused in the oil, the mixture is strained to remove the plant material, leaving behind the herb-infused oil. This oil is then combined with beeswax, which is melted into the oil to create a thicker, more stable form. The ratio of beeswax to oil determines the firmness of the final product; more beeswax results in a firmer ointment. Once the beeswax is fully melted and blended with the herbal oil, the mixture is poured into clean containers and allowed to cool and solidify.

How to Use: The finished cream or ointment can be applied topically to the skin, where it serves as a medium for the herbs' medicinal properties to be absorbed. These preparations are particularly useful for treating localized skin issues, such as wounds, burns, eczema, or rashes, providing both protective and healing benefits. The ointment's consistency allows it to stay on the skin longer, creating a barrier that supports skin repair and hydration.

(Poultices)

How to Make: This traditional method involves crushing fresh herbs or rehydrating dried herbs with a small amount of hot water to create a paste. The consistency of the paste should be thick enough to stick to the skin without dripping. The herbal paste is then spread directly onto a piece of clean cloth, gauze, or bandage.

How to Use: The cloth or gauze with the herbal paste is applied to the skin over the affected area, where the direct contact allows the therapeutic properties of the herbs to penetrate the skin and underlying tissues. The poultice can be secured with a wrap or bandage to keep it in place, often left on the skin for several hours or overnight. This method is effective for drawing out infections, reducing inflammation, and relieving pain. Poultices are particularly beneficial for abscesses, sprains, and deep-seated skin infections, allowing the active compounds in the herbs to be absorbed directly into the area needing treatment.

Compresses

How to Make: A compress is made by soaking a clean cloth or gauze in a hot or cold herbal infusion or decoction, depending on the condition being treated. The temperature of the compress can be tailored to the specific therapeutic need; hot compresses are generally used to relax muscles and increase blood flow, while cold compresses are used to reduce swelling and inflammation. To prepare, steep the chosen herbs in boiling water for a strong infusion or decoction, then soak the cloth in the liquid, ensuring it is fully saturated with the herbal extract.

How to Use: Wring out the excess liquid from the cloth and apply it directly to the affected area on the skin. The compress can be left in place for 15-30 minutes, or longer if needed, and can be reapplied several times a day. Compresses are versatile and can be used for a variety of issues, including muscle aches, bruises, inflammations, or even headaches, providing localized treatment that leverages the healing properties of herbs.

Aromatherapy & Essential Oils

How to Make: Creating essential oils for aromatherapy begins with selecting the right herbs, such as lavender for relaxation or peppermint for invigoration. The extraction process involves steam distillation, where the herbs are heated to release their aromatic oils. This can be achieved using a home distillation kit, where the plant material is placed in a chamber, steam circulates to extract the oils, and the mixture is then cooled to separate the oil and water. It's a meticulous process that captures the essence of the herb in its purest form, ensuring the therapeutic properties are preserved

How to Use: In aromatherapy, these essential oils are used to promote physical and emotional well-being. To use, dilute the concentrated oil with a carrier oil to prevent skin irritation before applying topically. For mental clarity or stress relief, add a few drops to a diffuser or inhaler. Alternatively, mix with bath salts for a soothing soak. When applied or inhaled, the aromatic molecules interact with the body's nasal sensory systems, influencing mood, energy levels, and overall health. Start with small quantities to gauge sensitivity and gradually adjust to suit personal preferences and therapeutic needs. To use essential herb oils topically, dilute with a carrier oil, like coconut or almond, and apply to the skin, targeting areas of tension or discomfort for relief.

Herbal Baths

How to Make: For a therapeutic herbal bath, create a strong infusion or decoction of your chosen herbs by steeping them in hot water for an extended period, which allows for a more concentrated extraction of their medicinal properties. After the herbs have steeped, strain the liquid to remove any plant material, then add this concentrated herbal solution to your bathwater. To enhance the therapeutic effects, consider adding Epsom salts, which are rich in magnesium, or a few drops of essential oils for additional aromatherapeutic benefits.

How to Use: Immerse yourself in the herbal bath for 15-30 minutes, allowing your body to absorb the herbal constituents through the skin. This method is particularly effective for soothing skin irritations, relieving muscle and joint pain, and promoting relaxation and stress relief. The warmth of the water helps to open pores and increase circulation, enhancing the absorption of the herbs' healing properties.

Steam Inhalation

How to Make: Begin by boiling a pot of water and then adding a generous amount of fresh or dried herbs. Allow the herbs to simmer in the boiling water for several minutes, which will enable them to release their essential oils and active compounds into the steam. Carefully pour the hot herbal water into a large bowl, ensuring it is stable and safe to use.

How to Use: Lean over the bowl and cover your head with a towel to create a tent that traps the steam. Inhale deeply for 5-10 minutes, allowing the herbal steam to enter the respiratory passages. This method is particularly effective for addressing respiratory issues, such as congestion, sinus infections, and cold symptoms. The direct inhalation of herbal steam can provide immediate relief for nasal and throat irritations and can help to open airways and alleviate respiratory discomfort.

Decoctions

How to Make: Decoctions are made by simmering the tougher parts of the plant, such as roots, barks, and seeds, in water for an extended period. This process helps to extract the water-soluble compounds that are more deeply embedded in the plant material. Place the plant parts in a pot, cover with water, and bring to a boil. Reduce the heat and simmer for 20-30 minutes, allowing the active ingredients to be released into the water.

How to Use: After simmering, strain the mixture to remove the solid plant materials, leaving behind the concentrated decoction. This can be consumed warm or allowed to cool, depending on the intended use. Decoctions are typically stronger than infusions and are used for their deeper, more systemic healing properties. They are particularly useful for chronic conditions, digestive issues, and as a supportive tonic for overall health. Because of their potency, decoctions can be used as a base for making syrups or added to other beverages to enhance flavor and medicinal value. They offer a robust way to deliver herbal benefits, especially when targeting specific internal systems or when a more concentrated dose of the herb's active compounds is needed for therapeutic effect.

Decoctions are particularly useful for deep-seated or chronic issues. By simmering the harder parts of the plant, you extract a broad spectrum of the plant's medicinal compounds, including those that are not easily released in teas or infusions. This method creates a potent remedy that can significantly aid the digestive system, support liver function, and boost the immune system. Decoctions can also be used externally as a wash for skin problems or as a compress for deep muscle or joint pain.

Syrups

How to Make: Syrups are made by simmering herbs with water to create a concentrated decoction. After straining out the plant material, the liquid is mixed with a sweetener, usually honey or sugar, until it dissolves into a thick syrup. You can infuse syrups with a variety of herbs depending on the desired therapeutic effect, such as thyme for respiratory issues or elderberry for immune support.

How to Use: Herbal syrups are taken orally and are especially effective for treating coughs, colds, and sore throats. They coat the throat and provide a soothing effect while delivering herbal benefits. Syrups can also be a delicious way to incorporate herbs into daily wellness routines, mixed into beverages or drizzled over food.

Gargles & Mouthwashes

How to Make: To create a gargle or mouthwash, steep the chosen herbs in hot water to form a strong infusion, then cool and strain the liquid. Antiseptic agents like salt, apple cider vinegar, or essential oils can be added to enhance the mouthwash's therapeutic properties.

How to Use: Gargling with herbal mouthwashes can relieve sore throats, reduce oral bacteria, and soothe mouth or gum irritations. Regular use of herbal mouthwashes can promote oral hygiene and prevent dental health issues.

Powders

How to Make: Dry the herbs thoroughly before grinding them into a fine powder. This can be done with a mortar and pestle or a mechanical grinder. The resulting powder should be stored in airtight containers to maintain its potency.

How to Use: Herbal powders are versatile and can be incorporated into capsules for easy ingestion, sprinkled on foods, or used in topical applications like pastes or poultices. They provide a concentrated dose of the herb's active ingredients and are beneficial for a wide range of health conditions.

Juices

How to Make: Fresh herbs, especially those with high water content, can be crushed or juiced to extract the liquid. This method preserves the raw, active enzymes and nutrients. To make juices from herbal plants, start by harvesting fresh, clean leaves or fruits. Chop them finely and place them in a blender with a little water. Blend until smooth, then strain the mixture through a fine mesh sieve or cheesecloth to remove any pulp. Add sweeteners or other flavors as desired, and enjoy the refreshing and nutritious herbal juice.

How to Use: Consuming fresh herbal juices provides an immediate influx of the plant's medicinal properties, supporting overall health and well-being. They are particularly useful for detoxification processes and can enhance vitality and energy levels.

Dosage and Administration:

Understanding how much and how often to take herbal medicines is key to getting the benefits you're looking for. It's like finding the sweet spot where the herb works its magic without going overboard. Think of it as tuning a guitar: too loose and there's no music, too tight and the string might snap.

Every herb is unique, so the right amount can vary a lot. For example, some herbs are super potent, so you only need a tiny bit, while others require more to do their thing. The form of the herb, like teas, tinctures, or capsules, also changes the amount you should use. Usually, a healthcare pro can guide you on the right dose.

Timing is another piece of the puzzle. Some herbs are taken as a "one-off" to help with sudden issues, like indigestion, while others are best used regularly to support ongoing health, like tonics for stress relief.

It's also crucial to consider your body's reaction. Everyone's different, so what works for one person might not be right for another. Starting with a lower dose and watching how your body responds can help you figure out the best amount for you. Plus, this approach can reduce the risk of side effects or herb interactions, especially if you're already taking other meds.

In short, using herbal medicine wisely means paying attention to how much, how often, and how you're taking it, always keeping in line with guidance from reliable sources or professionals in herbal medicine.

Safety and Precautions:

Navigating the world of herbal medicine can be incredibly rewarding, but it's crucial to be aware of potential side effects and interactions with medications. Herbs, just like pharmaceutical drugs, contain active compounds that can affect our bodies in various ways.

Starting with side effects, most herbs are safe when used appropriately. However, individual reactions can vary. For example, while chamomile is generally known for its calming effects, some people might experience allergic reactions, especially if they are allergic to related plants like ragweed. It's vital to start with small doses to monitor how your body responds and to recognize any adverse effects early on.

Interaction with medications is another critical area. Herbs can either amplify or diminish the effects of pharmaceutical drugs. For instance, St. John's Wort is notorious for interacting with a wide range of medications, including antidepressants and birth control pills, often reducing their effectiveness. If you're taking any medication, it's essential to consult with a healthcare provider before starting any herbal regimen. They can advise you on potential interactions based on your specific medications and health conditions.

Knowing when to avoid certain herbs is equally important. Some herbs are not recommended in specific situations, such as pregnancy or while breastfeeding. For example, pregnant women are often advised to avoid herbs like goldenseal and wormwood due to their potent active compounds that can affect the pregnancy. Additionally, conditions like high blood pressure or diabetes might require you to steer clear of certain herbs that could exacerbate these conditions.

While herbs offer a natural way to support health, they must be used with knowledge and caution. Always do your research, consult with professionals, and listen to your body. By being informed about potential side effects, medication interactions, and contraindications, you can make safer choices in your herbal medicine journey, ensuring that you reap the benefits without unnecessary risks.

Herbal Combination Formulas:

Deciding which herbal formulas to make can seem daunting, but it's all about matching your health needs with the right herbs. Here's a step-by-step guide to get you started and ensure you craft effective herbal remedies.

1. Identify Your Health Goal

Start by pinpointing exactly what you want to address. Is it a recurring headache, digestive issues, or maybe stress? Your health goal will guide which herbs you select. Research herbs known for treating your specific ailment. Books, reputable online resources, or consulting with an herbalist can provide valuable insights.

2. Choose Your Herbs

Once you've identified your health goal, select herbs that have a history of treating that condition. For example, if you're targeting sleep problems, herbs like valerian or chamomile might be your go-to. But remember, it's not just about picking one herb. Consider how different herbs can work together for a more comprehensive treatment.

3. Understand Herb Interactions

Before mixing herbs, understand their interactions. Some herbs amplify each other's effects, while others might counteract them. For instance, combining calming herbs can enhance their soothing properties, but mixing stimulating herbs with sedatives could negate the benefits.

4. Decide on the Formula Type

Herbal formulas can be teas, tinctures, capsules, or topical applications like salves and creams. The choice depends on your preference and the best method for administering the herbs' benefits. Teas might be ideal for digestion aids, while tinctures or capsules could be better for long-term conditions like joint health.

5. Crafting Your Formula

For teas or infusions, blend dried herbs in proportions that align with their strength and your goal. Use a scale for accuracy, mixing them thoroughly. For tinctures, fill a jar one-third to one-half with dried herbs, then cover completely with your alcohol or vinegar. Seal and label the jar, storing it in a cool, dark place, shaking it daily for 4 to 6 weeks.

For a topical application, like a salve, gently heat the herbs in a carrier oil to extract their properties, strain, then mix with beeswax until melted and pour into containers to solidify.

6. Test and Adjust

After making your formula, test it to see how your body reacts. It's okay if it's not perfect on the first try; adjusting is part of the process.

Maybe you need to tweak the herb ratios or switch the administration method. Pay attention to how you feel and adjust accordingly.

7. Documentation
Keep detailed notes of the herbs, amounts, and methods used. This record-keeping is invaluable for refining your formulas and tracking what works best for you.

Final Thoughts... In creating herbal formulas, patience and experimentation are key. Start simple, with two or three herbs, and gradually build complexity as you gain confidence and knowledge. Tailor your creations to your body's responses and preferences, refining over time to perfect your personal herbal pharmacy.

By following these steps, you'll develop a methodical approach to crafting herbal remedies that are specifically tailored to your needs, ensuring you use the right herbs in the right way to promote health and well-being.

Customizing Remedies:
Herbal medicine shines when it's personalized. Just like a custom suit or outfit is tailored to fit your measurements perfectly, herbal treatments can be customized to suit your unique needs. Here's how to do it right:

- **Age Matters:** Kids, adults, and the elderly all process herbs differently. Children often need milder, less concentrated doses. On the flip side, older adults might have slower metabolism rates, affecting how they process herbs. Always adjust dosages according to age and, when in doubt, consult with a herbalist or healthcare provider.

- **Body Constitution:** Personalizing herbal medicine ensures it fits your unique physical and health profile perfectly. Age is crucial, as children and the elderly metabolize herbs differently, necessitating adjusted dosages. Your body's constitution, whether influenced by genetic makeup or environmental factors, dictates your herbal needs, highlighting the importance of matching remedies to individual traits and conditions. This approach maximizes the herbs' benefits while minimizing risks, creating a safer and more effective herbal treatment plan.

- **Specific Health Conditions:** Customizing herbal treatments to specific health issues is essential. If you're battling insomnia, certain herbs could help you sleep better. However, if you also suffer from high blood pressure, it's important to choose herbs that can effectively manage both conditions without adverse reactions. This careful selection ensures that the herbal regimen not only targets the problems but also harmonizes with your overall health, avoiding complications..

- **Lifestyle and Environment:** Your daily routine and environment play a significant role. If you're living in a polluted city, herbs that support lung health can be helpful. Similarly, if your job is high-stress, adaptogenic herbs that help manage stress levels could be integral to your herbal regimen.

By considering these factors, you can create an herbal treatment plan that's as unique as you are. This personalized approach not only enhances the effectiveness of the herbs but also minimizes potential side effects, ensuring that your journey with herbal medicine is both safe and beneficial.

Labeling and Documentation:

Documenting your herbal remedy adventures is a smart move. Here's how to do it effectively:

- **Ingredients:** List all the herbs and additional components you use in your mixtures. This will help you keep track of what works and identify any reactions or allergies. Think of it as your personal herbal recipe book that you can refine over time.
- **Dates:** Note when you make and use your remedies. This timeline can be a lifesaver when trying to figure out which treatments are most effective during different seasons or health conditions. It's like having a diary that tracks your herbal health journey.
- **Usage Instructions:** Write down how to prepare and use each remedy. This could include the amount of herb used, boiling times for teas, or the duration for applying a topical ointment. It's your personalized user manual for natural health care.

Keeping these records isn't just about organization; it's about equipping yourself with knowledge. You'll be able to see patterns, understand what influences your well-being, and make informed decisions about your health. Plus, if you ever want to share your herbal wisdom with others, you'll have detailed notes to pass on. It's a great way to contribute to the community of herbal enthusiasts and help others on their path to natural wellness

Storage and Preservation:

Storing herbs correctly is like keeping your favorite snacks fresh – you want them tasty and effective when you're ready to use them. Here's how to ensure your herbs retain their potency, flavor, and medicinal properties.

Drying Herbs

Drying is one of the oldest and most efficient ways to preserve herbs. The goal is to remove moisture while keeping the essential oils (that's where all the goodness lies) intact. Hang bunches of herbs upside down in a warm, dry place with good air circulation, away from direct sunlight. An attic or a pantry works well. Wait until the leaves are crumbly, usually a few weeks, then store them in an airtight container.

If you're in a hurry, an oven or dehydrator can speed up the process. Set the temperature low, around 95-115°F. Keep a close eye on them; herbs can lose their vibrant color and potency if overheated.

Freezing Herbs

Freezing is fantastic for preserving the flavor and therapeutic properties of herbs. Wash and pat the herbs dry, chop them finely, and spread them on a baking sheet to freeze individually. Once frozen, transfer them to a freezer-safe bag or container. This method keeps them separate and easy to measure for later use.

Another great trick is to freeze herbs in ice cube trays with water or oil. Pop out a cube whenever you need a flavor boost in your cooking or a base for your herbal preparations.

Choosing the Right Containers

The right container can make a big difference in how well your herbs are preserved. Glass jars with airtight lids are ideal. They protect herbs from moisture, light, and air, which can degrade their quality over time. Dark-colored glass is even better, especially for light-sensitive herbs.

Plastic is okay for short-term storage, but it's not the best for long-term since it can interact with the herbs and affect their flavor and potency. Metal containers are another option, but make sure they're food-grade and don't react with the herbs.

Label and Date

Your containers should always list the herb name, and the date of storage. It helps keep track of freshness and ensures you're using herbs at their peak potency. Storing herbs properly isn't just about extending their shelf life; it's about preserving their essence and ensuring they're effective and beneficial when you need them.

Purchasing Herbs from Outside Sources

When exploring the world of herbalism, it's crucial to think about where your herbs come from and how they're gathered. Ethical sourcing and sustainable practices aren't just fancy terms; they're actions that protect our planet and ensure the plants we rely on will be around for future generations.

First up, let's talk about ethical sourcing. This means buying herbs from suppliers who harvest plants responsibly. It's like choosing fair-trade coffee or chocolate. You're supporting a system that looks after the people who nurture and collect the herbs.

Then there's sustainability, a big word with a simple concept: use resources in a way that doesn't deplete them. In herbalism, this means harvesting herbs in a manner that allows the plant population to regenerate. Overharvesting is a real problem, especially for popular herbs that are in high demand. By choosing sustainably harvested herbs, you're helping to ensure that these plants can continue to grow in their natural habitats.

Why does this matter to you? Well, besides the feel-good factor of doing the right thing, these practices directly impact the quality of the herbs you use and, by extension, the effectiveness of your herbal remedies. Healthy plants from a balanced ecosystem make for potent remedies. Plus, by supporting ethical and sustainable practices, you're contributing to a healthier environment and a more equal and harmonious society.

So, when you pick up that next batch of purchased herbs, take a moment to consider their journey to you. Choosing ethically sourced and sustainably harvested herbs is a win-win for you, the community, and the earth.

7. Culinary Options

Pairing Herbs with Foods for Flavor and Health

Pairing herbs with foods is not just about adding flavor; it's about creating a symphony of taste and wellness that resonates with every bite. This culinary strategy enhances dishes with herbs' unique flavors and medicinal properties, leading to a holistic dining experience. It's about striking the right balance, where the herb enhances the food's natural flavor without overpowering it.

Mint, known for its refreshing flavor, is excellent in salads, drinks, or desserts, aiding in digestion and offering a cooling sensation. Rosemary, with its robust aroma, is not only ideal for roasting meats but also offers cognitive and circulatory benefits. On the other hand, basil, with its sweet and peppery essence, can transform a simple tomato sauce while providing anti-inflammatory and antibacterial advantages.

Thyme, another versatile herb, can be used in marinades, soups, and stews, imparting a subtle earthy flavor while supporting respiratory and immune health. Similarly, oregano, with its bold and peppery taste, can be sprinkled on pizzas, pasta, or salads, adding not just flavor but also antioxidants that support overall health.

Herbs like cilantro can be used in salsas, rice dishes, or as garnishes, providing a fresh, tangy flavor and detoxifying benefits. Incorporating lavender into baked goods or teas can create soothing and stress-relieving culinary experiences. It's these thoughtful combinations that elevate everyday meals into nourishing culinary creations.

Ultimately, the integration of herbs into your diet should be an enjoyable and health-conscious endeavor. It's about making each meal an opportunity to nourish your body and delight your taste buds. By embracing the art of pairing herbs with foods, you create a culinary landscape where flavor and health coexist harmoniously, leading to a richer, more satisfying eating experience.

Creative Uses of Herbs in Beverages

Herbs bring a world of flavor and health benefits to beverages as well, offering an array of possibilities for quenching thirst in the most nourishing way. From the calming properties of chamomile tea to the digestive benefits of ginger-infused drinks, herbs can transform beverages into wellness elixirs. Take, for example, mint, a versatile herb that can be used in everything from herbal teas to refreshing cocktails like mojitos, offering both a cool flavor and digestive aid.

Lemon balm, with its mild lemon scent, is fantastic in iced teas or lemonades, providing a soothing effect that can reduce stress and anxiety. Similarly, the subtle floral notes of lavender can be infused into lemonades or cocktails, creating drinks that not only tantalize the taste buds but also calm the mind.

For a more invigorating experience, rosemary can be steeped in hot water or mixed into cocktails for its unique, pine-like flavor and its ability to boost memory and concentration. Similarly, thyme can be used in teas or mixed drinks, bringing a unique earthy flavor and aiding in respiratory and immune health.

Herbs like basil and cilantro can be crushed and added to drinks for a burst of flavor. Basil, with its sweet and peppery taste, is excellent in homemade lemonades or infused waters, promoting digestive health and providing anti-inflammatory benefits. Cilantro, known for its detoxifying properties, adds a fresh, tangy element to juices and smoothies.

Moreover, herbal beverages can be a delightful way to introduce the healing properties of lesser-known herbs like echinacea, known for its immune-boosting properties, in teas or warm drinks, especially during cold and flu season.

Incorporating herbs into beverages is not just about adding flavor; it's about enhancing the health benefits of your hydration choices. With each herb offering unique flavors and medicinal properties, the possibilities are endless, allowing for a creative and healthful approach to everyday drinks. This integration of herbs into beverages is a testament to their versatility and power, making every sip a delicious step towards better health.

Creating Seasonings, Spices and Condiments

Creating these additions from your own herb garden can transform your culinary experience, offering a fresher, healthier, and more personalized approach to flavoring your dishes. Utilizing herbs such as basil, oregano, and thyme, allows you to create unique blends that are not only delicious but also packed with health benefits.

The process of making your own seasonings starts with harvesting the right parts of the herb plants at the optimal time, usually just before they flower, when their oils and flavors are most potent. For dried seasonings, you can air-dry or use a dehydrator to remove moisture from the herbs, ensuring they retain their aroma and medicinal properties. Once dried, the herbs can be ground into powder or left whole, depending on the intended use.

To make spice blends, combine ground versions of compatible herbs, such as oregano, thyme, and rosemary, adjusting the ratios to suit your taste. These blends can be stored in airtight containers and used to season a variety of dishes, from meats and vegetables to soups and sauces, offering a burst of flavor and a boost of antioxidants.

Creating condiments like herb-infused oils and vinegars is another fantastic way to preserve and use your garden herbs. Simply submerge fresh herbs in olive oil or vinegar and let them infuse for several weeks in a cool, dark place. The result is a flavorful condiment that can be used to dress salads, marinate meats, or add a finishing touch to dishes, providing both the nuanced flavors of the herbs and their health-enhancing properties.

For those who enjoy a bit of heat, making chili oils with herbs like oregano or rosemary can add a spicy kick to your meals. Similarly, crafting herb-based rubs for barbecue or roasting can elevate the taste of your proteins and vegetables, infusing them with complex, aromatic flavors.

The joy of creating your own seasonings, spices, and condiments lies in the ability to tailor them to your taste preferences and health needs. For instance, if you are looking to improve digestion, incorporating herbs like fennel or mint into your seasonings can be beneficial. Moreover, homemade creations often lack the preservatives and artificial additives found in store-bought products, making them a healthier choice.

Developing a collection of homemade seasonings, spices, and condiments from your herb garden not only enhances the flavors of your cooking but also contributes to a healthier, more sustainable lifestyle. It allows you to control the quality of your ingredients!

8. Special Focus on Mental Well-Being

Herbs for Stress, Anxiety, and Sleep Disorders:

Understanding and applying the world of herbal remedies can be a game-changer for managing stress, anxiety, and sleep issues. Imagine having a natural toolkit at your fingertips to help soothe your mind and promote restful sleep. Let's look at how certain herbs can be your allies in achieving better mental well-being and sleep quality.

First up, let's talk about stress. It's always an unwelcome guest. Herbs like ashwagandha come into play here. Known for its adaptogenic properties, meaning it helps your body manage stress more effectively. Think of it as helping your body's stress response system become more resilient, kind of like upgrading your internal stress-handling software.

Anxiety, on the other hand, is like a constant buzz of worry in the background. Herbs like chamomile and lemon balm are fantastic for dialing down this noise. Chamomile, often enjoyed as a calming tea, works wonders in easing nervous tension and promoting relaxation. Lemon balm, with its mild sedative effect, can help reduce anxiety and bring a sense of calm.

Now, let's move on to sleep disorders. If counting sheep isn't cutting it for you, consider herbs like valerian root and lavender. Valerian root is often used as a natural treatment for insomnia. It's like nature's version of hitting the snooze button on your brain's overactivity, helping you drift off to sleep. Lavender, with its soothing scent, is excellent for creating a relaxing bedtime atmosphere. Using it in an essential oil diffuser or in a pillow spray can help prepare your mind and body for sleep.

Remember, while these herbs are helpful, they're part of a larger wellness picture. Incorporating them into a routine that includes healthy sleep hygiene, regular exercise, and good nutrition will offer the best results. Also, it's crucial to remember that what works for one person might not work for another. It's all about finding the right balance and combination that works for you.

Finally, before you start using herbal remedies, it's wise to consult with a healthcare provider if you're already taking medications or have underlying health conditions. Herbs are powerful, and it's important to use them mindfully to ensure they benefit your health without causing unintended side effects.

Incorporating Therapeutic Gardening Practices into Daily Life:

Gardening isn't just about growing plants; it can be a therapeutic road that nurtures both your garden and your well-being. Imagine stepping into your backyard, balcony, or even a windowsill garden, and feeling a sense of calm wash over you. That's the magic of therapeutic gardening! It's about creating a green space that becomes your sanctuary, a place where stress fades and peace prevails.

- **Connecting with Nature:** Gardening allows you to get your hands dirty, literally grounding you as you connect with the earth. This hands-on interaction with soil and plants can boost your mood and decrease stress levels. It's like nature's way of giving you a big, calming hug.
- **Mindfulness and Presence:** Focusing on the simple tasks of planting, watering, and tending to your garden can help anchor you in the present moment. This mindfulness practice can be a powerful antidote to the fast-paced digital world,

offering a pause to just be and breathe among your leafy companions.

- **Physical Activity:** Gardening involves bending, digging, planting, and walking, which are great physical activities that can improve your fitness. It's a gentle way to keep your body moving, enjoy some fresh air, and soak up a bit of sunshine for that vital vitamin D.

- **Nurturing Growth:** Watching something you planted grow and thrive is incredibly rewarding. It's a reminder of the cycles of life and growth, teaching patience and care. Each sprout and bloom can be a metaphor for personal growth and success.

- **Sensory Stimulation:** Gardens are a feast for the senses. The scent of fresh herbs, the sound of rustling leaves, the sight of colorful flowers, and the taste of home-grown veggies can all enhance your sensory experience and contribute to a feeling of well-being.

- **Creating a Habitat:** Your garden can become a sanctuary for birds, bees, butterflies, and other wildlife, adding another layer of satisfaction to your gardening efforts. It's rewarding to know you're contributing to the local ecosystem, providing a haven for these creatures.

- **Therapeutic Design:** Consider creating a garden layout that encourages relaxation and reflection. Incorporate elements like water features for their soothing sounds, or create a cozy nook with a bench where you can sit and enjoy the fruits of your labor.

- **Cultivating Community:** Gardening can be a communal activity. Sharing your space with friends, family, or community members can strengthen bonds and foster a sense of belonging. Community gardens are fantastic for connecting with neighbors and fellow garden enthusiasts.

- **Emotional Healing:** There's something profoundly healing about caring for plants. It can be a form of emotional expression and release, helping to manage feelings of sadness, anxiety, or loneliness.

Incorporating therapeutic gardening into your daily life means more than just tending to plants; it's about nurturing your soul, enhancing your physical health, and creating a peaceful retreat from the stresses of everyday life. Whether you have acres of land or just a few pots on a windowsill, gardening can be tailored to fit your space and lifestyle, bringing a piece of nature's therapy into your daily routine.

Part IV
Advanced Herbal Practices

9. The Urban Herbalist's Guide

Overcoming Space Limitations:

Living in the city, or an apartment, or any urban setting really doesn't mean you have to forgo the joys of gardening. Even in the heart of the city, you can cultivate a lush herbal haven right in your own space. Whether it's a tiny balcony, a sunny windowsill, or a cozy indoor nook, there are myriad ways to grow and nurture herbs. This section will show you how to transform even the smallest urban area into a productive and serene green space, bringing nature's bounty into your urban life.

Balconies

1. Assess Your Space: First, take a look at your balcony. How much space do you have? Which direction does it face? Herbs love sunlight, so a south-facing balcony is ideal, but many herbs can still thrive with partial sunlight on east or west-facing balconies.

2. Choose Your Herbs: Decide which herbs you want to grow based on your cooking preferences and the climate. Hardy herbs like rosemary, thyme, and sage are great for beginners and can withstand more varied conditions. If you have a bit more sunlight and warmth, try basil, cilantro, or mint.

3. Get the Right Containers: Pots or containers with good drainage are crucial. Herbs don't like soggy roots, so make sure each pot has drainage holes. If space is tight, consider vertical gardening solutions like tiered planters or hanging pots.

4. Use Quality Soil: Herbs thrive in well-draining soil. Use a potting mix designed for containers, which will retain moisture without getting waterlogged. Mixing in a little compost can provide extra nutrients for your herbs.

5. Planting: You can start herbs from seeds or buy young plants from a nursery. If starting from seeds, plant them according to the depth and spacing recommendations on the packet. For young plants, gently remove them from their containers, loosen the roots, and plant them in your pots, making sure they're at the same depth they were in their nursery pots.

6. Watering: Herbs generally like to be watered regularly but allow the soil to dry out slightly between watering. Over-watering can lead to root rot, so it's better to water less frequently than too often.

7. Feeding: Use a balanced, water-soluble fertilizer every few weeks to ensure your herbs have all the nutrients they need, especially if you're harvesting them regularly.

8. Regular Maintenance: Check your herbs daily for signs of pests or disease. Regular pruning will encourage bushier growth and prevent the plants from becoming leggy.

9. Harvesting: Begin to harvest your herbs once they're established. Regular picking encourages new growth and can prevent the plants from going to seed too early.

By following these steps, you can successfully grow a range of herbs on your urban balcony, bringing a bit of greenery and freshness to your city-living.

Windowsills

Growing herbs on a windowsill is a fantastic way to bring a bit of nature into your urban home and have fresh flavors at your fingertips. Here's how to start your windowsill herb garden:

1. Evaluate Your Window: Check which direction your window faces. South-facing windows are best for herbs as they get the most light. East or west-facing windows also work, but north-facing windows may need additional grow lights.

2. Select Your Herbs: Choose herbs that thrive in limited space and can grow well indoors. Compact herbs like basil, chives, parsley, and mint are ideal for windowsill gardening.

3. Pick the Right Pots: Use pots or containers with good drainage holes to prevent water from sitting at the bottom. Consider narrow, long planters that fit well on the windowsill or individual pots for different herbs.

4. Use Quality Potting Mix: Fill your containers with a high-quality potting mix designed for indoor plants. This will ensure good drainage and provide essential nutrients to your herbs.

5. Plant Your Herbs: You can start from seeds or purchase small herb plants from a garden center. If using seeds, plant them according to the packet's instructions. For seedlings, ensure they're planted at the same depth as their previous container.

6. Watering Wisely: Herbs don't like to be too wet. Water them when the top inch of soil feels dry to the touch. Be cautious not to over-water, especially in lower light conditions.

7. Providing Light: Herbs need plenty of light. Aim for at least 6 hours of sunlight per day. If natural light is insufficient, supplement with a grow light to ensure your herbs thrive.

8. Feeding Your Herbs: Use a liquid fertilizer every 4-6 weeks, but avoid over-fertilizing, which can weaken the plants and dilute the flavor of the herbs.

9. Pruning and Harvesting: Regularly pinch back or trim your herbs to encourage fuller, bushier plants. Harvest as needed, but never remove more than one-third of the plant at a time to allow it to recover.

10. Monitoring for Pests: Keep an eye out for pests like aphids or spider mites. If you spot any, treat your plants with a natural insecticide or a mild soap solution.

By following these steps, you can create a lush, productive herb garden right on your windowsill, adding freshness and greenery to your urban living space.

Indoor Gardens

Creating an indoor garden with artificial lighting is a fantastic solution for growing herbs year-round, regardless of natural sunlight availability. With the right setup, you can cultivate a flourishing herb garden indoors, adding fresh flavors to your cooking and greenery to your space.

Starting Off Right

Begin by selecting a space in your home that can accommodate your indoor garden. It could be a corner of your kitchen, a dedicated room, or even a shelf. The key is to choose a location where your plants won't be in the way but can still be easily accessed for care and harvesting.

Choosing Your Lighting

Artificial lights (more on this in next section) are crucial for indoor gardening, especially in areas lacking natural sunlight. LED grow lights are ideal because they emit a spectrum of light that herbs need for photosynthesis and are energy-efficient. Ensure the lights cover the entire growing area evenly and can be adjusted as plants grow.

Selecting Herbs

Opt for herbs that thrive in indoor conditions, such as basil, mint, oregano, parsley, chives, and thyme. These herbs generally do well under artificial lighting and don't require as much direct sunlight as some other plants.

Containers and Soil

Use containers with good drainage holes to prevent waterlogging, which can lead to root rot. Fill them with a high-quality potting mix that is well-draining yet retains enough moisture to nourish the roots. Adding a layer of gravel or pebbles at the bottom of each pot can enhance drainage.

Planting

You can start your herbs from seeds or buy young plants from a nursery. If starting from seeds, plant them according to the depth and spacing recommendations on the seed packet. For young plants, always make sure they are planted at the same depth they were in their nursery containers.

Lighting Schedule

Herbs need around 14-16 hours of artificial light each day to mimic natural sunlight. Use a timer for your grow lights to maintain a consistent light cycle, providing your herbs with the regularity they need for optimal growth.

Watering

Herbs prefer the soil to be slightly dry between watering. Check the soil regularly; if the top inch is dry, it's time to water. Over-watering can be as harmful as under-watering, so ensure your containers allow excess water to drain away.

Nutrition

Feed your herbs with a balanced, water-soluble fertilizer every four weeks, but be careful not to over-fertilize, as this can harm plant growth and affect the taste of your herbs.

Pruning and Harvesting

Regular pruning encourages bushier, healthier growth and prevents herbs from becoming leggy. Harvest your herbs by snipping off what you need, but never take more than one-third of the plant at once, to allow it to recover and continue growing.

Temperature and Humidity

Most herbs prefer temperatures between 65-75°F (18-24°C). Avoid placing them near drafts, radiators, or air conditioning units, which can cause temperature fluctuations. If your indoor air is dry, consider using a humidifier or placing a water tray near the growing area to increase humidity.

Pest Management

Inspect your herbs regularly for signs of pests. If you find any, isolate the affected plant to prevent spread and treat it with a natural pesticide or a homemade solution like soapy water.

Troubleshooting

If your herbs are not thriving, assess their growing conditions. Yellowing leaves might indicate over-watering or poor drainage, while leggy (or too stemmy) growth suggests inadequate light. Adjust your care routine accordingly to address these issues.

Expanding Your Garden

As you become more experienced, consider diversifying your indoor herb garden. Experiment with different herb varieties or introduce companion plants that can coexist beneficially.

Enjoy Your Harvest

The best part of indoor gardening is the harvest. Use your fresh herbs to enhance your meals, make teas, or as aromatic additions to your home.

By following these detailed steps, you can successfully grow a vibrant and productive herb garden indoors. It's a rewarding way to bring a piece of nature into your home and enjoy the fresh, flavorful benefits of your own hand-grown herbs.

Artificial Indoor Lighting

Growing herbs indoors using artificial lighting involves understanding various lighting options, their features, and how to implement them effectively. Here's a comprehensive guide:

Types of Artificial Lighting

- **Fluorescent Lights:** Ideal for herbs due to their cool temperature. They come in tubes or compact bulbs (CFLs). Standard fluorescent bulbs are suitable for low-light herbs like mint and parsley, while high-output fluorescents and T5 bulbs are better for high-light herbs like basil and thyme.
- **LED Lights:** Highly efficient and long-lasting, LEDs emit a full spectrum of light, mimicking natural sunlight. They generate less heat and are available in various spectrums and intensities to suit different stages of plant growth.
- **High-Intensity Discharge (HID) Lights:** Including Metal Halide (MH) and High-Pressure Sodium (HPS) lamps, HIDs are powerful and effective for larger indoor gardens. MH lamps support vegetative growth with their cool, blue spectrum, while HPS lamps, emitting a warm, red spectrum, are better for flowering and fruiting stages.
- **Incandescent Lights:** (traditional filament bulbs) Generally not recommended for growing herbs as they emit more heat and less suitable light spectrum, which can harm plant growth.

Choosing the Right Lighting

- **Space:** The size of your growing area will determine the intensity and coverage needed from your grow lights. Larger spaces may require more powerful lights or a combination of lights to ensure even coverage.
- **Budget:** LEDs tend to be more expensive initially but offer savings in the long run due to lower energy consumption and replacement costs. Fluorescent and HID lights can be less

expensive upfront but may cost more over time in energy and maintenance.

- **Ease of Use:** Consider fixtures that are easy to install, adjust, and maintain. Many grow lights come with adjustable stands or hanging systems to change the light height as plants grow.

Purchasing Your Grow Lights

When buying grow lights, consider retailers that specialize in gardening and hydroponic supplies, as they can provide expert advice tailored to your specific needs. Online retailers offer a wide range of options with customer reviews that can help guide your decision. Local gardening centers or hydroponic stores are also valuable resources for finding high-quality lights and getting personalized advice.

Setting Up Your Lighting System

- **Installation:** The method of installing your lights will depend on their type and your space. Common setups include hanging lights from the ceiling, mounting them on walls, or using free standing lamp stands. Ensure your lights are securely attached and positioned to evenly distribute light across all plants.
- **Height and Positioning:** The ideal height of lights above your plants varies with the light intensity and plant type. Generally, LEDs should be 12-24 inches above the plants, fluorescents about 6-12 inches, and HIDs around 24-36 inches, adjusting as plants grow to prevent burning or insufficient light exposure.
- **Lighting Schedule:** Herbs typically need 14-16 hours of light per day. Use a timer to regulate the light/dark cycle, mimicking natural conditions and promoting healthy plant growth.

- **Monitoring Growth:** Observe your plants regularly for signs of too much or too little light (e.g., weak, leggy growth or scorched leaves) and adjust height and duration accordingly.
- **Reflective Surfaces:** Increase light efficiency by placing reflective materials like mylar, white paint, or aluminum foil around the garden area to reflect light back onto the plants.
- **Ventilation:** While LEDs and fluorescents generate less heat, HID lights can get very hot; ensure your indoor garden has good air circulation to prevent heat buildup. Use fans or ventilation systems as necessary.
- **Safety:** Keep electrical connections safe from water and ensure that your lighting setup is secure to prevent accidents.

Maintenance and Troubleshooting

- Regularly clean the light bulbs or tubes to remove dust and ensure maximum light output.
- Replace bulbs as per the manufacturer's recommendation or if you notice a significant decrease in light intensity.
- If plants show signs of distress, reassess their light requirements, as different herbs have varying needs for light intensity and duration.

Conclusion - Effective use of artificial lighting can make indoor herb gardening a successful and fulfilling endeavor. LED lights are generally the best option for indoor herbs, offering energy efficiency, longevity, and a suitable light spectrum. By carefully setting up your lighting system, maintaining an appropriate light schedule, and monitoring plant growth, you can cultivate healthy, vibrant herbs indoors, regardless of natural sunlight availability. This approach enables year-round cultivation of your favorite herbs, adding freshness and greenery to your urban living space.

10. Growing Herbs in Limited Spaces

Vertical Gardening utilizes wall planters, trellises, or hanging pots, allowing the cultivation of various herbs in a space-efficient manner. This method is ideal for urban environments where horizontal space is limited, enabling a lush, green facade or indoor garden wall that brings a touch of nature to the urban jungle.

Rooftop Gardens transform underutilized flat rooftops into productive green spaces, providing ample sunlight and fresh air for a wide range of herbs. This approach not only maximizes the use of available space but also contributes to urban biodiversity, creating a haven for pollinators and beneficial insects in city settings.

Hydroponic Systems offer a soil-less, water-based method for growing herbs, utilizing nutrient-rich solutions to feed the plants. This technique is perfect for indoor environments, as it reduces the need for large outdoor spaces, minimizes pest problems, and allows for year-round cultivation regardless of external weather conditions.

Aquaponics combines aquaculture (raising fish) and hydroponics (growing plants in water) in a symbiotic environment. In this system, fish waste provides organic food for the plants, and the plants naturally filter the water for the fish. It's a sustainable, eco-friendly method that can be implemented indoors, making it suitable for urban dwellers interested in both herb gardening and fish farming.

Terrarium Gardening involves creating miniature ecosystems within glass containers, ideal for small, humidity-loving plants. This method allows for the creation of controlled, self-sustaining environments that can add decorative greenery to indoor spaces while requiring minimal maintenance.

Kitchen Counter Gardens make use of small containers or hydroponic kits placed on kitchen counters, enabling the growth of herbs within arm's reach. This method is perfect for culinary enthusiasts who value the convenience of fresh herbs for cooking and garnishing, enhancing both the flavor of dishes and the aesthetics of your kitchen space.

Rail Planters attach to the balcony or stair rails, offering a space-saving solution for growing herbs without encroaching on valuable floor or ground area. These planters are perfect for adding greenery to elevated spaces, enhancing the visual appeal of balconies and stairways while providing easy access to fresh herbs.

Pocket Gardens utilize hanging pocket organizers or fabric wall planters, turning vertical surfaces into lush, plant-filled areas. Each pocket can be filled with soil and planted with herbs, creating a living tapestry that is both functional and decorative, ideal for maximizing the use of vertical space in confined areas.

Gutter Gardens repurpose old gutters into horizontal planters that can be mounted on exterior walls or fences. This method is excellent for growing herbs that require good drainage and can be easily accessed for harvesting. Gutter gardens are a creative and efficient way to utilize narrow spaces for gardening in urban environments.

Mason Jar Gardens involve growing herbs in mason jars filled with potting mix, which can be placed on indoor shelves or hung in front of windows to receive natural light. This approach combines rustic charm with practicality, offering a compact and visually appealing way to grow herbs indoors.

11. From Urban Garden to Urban Health

Herbal Gardening: Improved Mental Health

Urban herbal gardening is not just a green touch to your city space; it's a real boost to your mental and physical health. Think of it as creating a mini oasis among the sometimes hectic world we all live in, where every herb like rosemary or thyme you grow brings a piece of nature's calm to your life. It's like crafting your little sanctuary, where the simple acts of planting and tending to herbs can melt away stress and bring a sense of achievement.

Imagine stepping onto your balcony or looking at your windowsill, greeted by the vibrant greens and aromatic scents of fresh herbs. This small garden is not just pleasing to the eyes but also a treasure trove of organic goodies for your kitchen, making your meals healthier and more flavorful.

But there's more to it than just the physical benefits. Tending to these plants can be a peaceful retreat from the urban rush, helping to soothe your mind and reduce anxiety. Plus, this green hobby can connect you with like-minded gardeners in your community, adding a dash of social wellness to your life.

Urban herbal gardening merges nature with city life, enhancing your living space, promoting health, and keeping you connected to nature. This practice proves that, even in the fast-paced urban environment, there's space to prosper alongside your green friends, blending green serenity with metropolitan vitality.

Community Benefits and Social Features of Urban Herbalism

Urban herbalism is about fostering a sense of community and connection. In city landscapes, where green spaces are often limited, creating herbal gardens can bring neighbors together, bridging the gap between nature and urban life. These communal gardens become more than just plots of land; they're gathering spots where people share knowledge, seeds, and harvests, sometimes even creating relationships and mutual support.

Moreover, urban herbalism can ignite conversations about sustainability and environmental stewardship, inspiring more city dwellers to engage in green practices. It's a stepping stone towards a more health-conscious and eco-friendly urban life, where people feel connected to their environment and each other. Through the simple act of growing herbs, urbanites can cultivate a community spirit, making the city a warmer, more welcoming place.

Part V
100 BEST Herbs to Grow

12. Herbal Plant Profiles

Ease to Grow Reference:

Low Maintenance 1-3: Plants in this category require minimal care, thriving with basic watering and occasional feeding. They are resilient, adaptable to various conditions, and rarely need pruning or specialized treatment.

Medium Maintenance 4-6: These plants need regular care, including consistent watering, feeding, and pruning. They may have specific light and soil preferences and could be more sensitive to environmental changes.

High Maintenance 7-9: High-maintenance plants demand attentive care, precise watering, specific humidity levels, and frequent feeding. They often require pest and disease management and are less tolerant of neglect.

Expert Level 10: These plants require expert care, with exacting requirements for climate, watering, feeding, and pruning. They often need controlled environments and are susceptible to stress and diseases, requiring constant monitoring and specialized knowledge.

This is a growing book!

Each of the next 100 plants has its own live QR code with color photos. The first 6 pictures we've included (simply scan with your phone or device to view), all others have been added from readers like you!

We encourage you to send us any photo of plants you are currently growing, or in any way using them (plus a little about what we are seeing). We'll then add your color photos to become part of this 'Growing Book'.

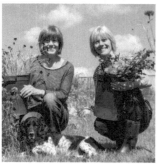
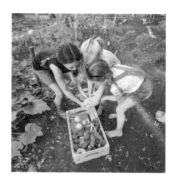
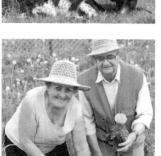
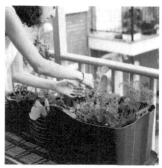

By submitting your photos, you grant us the right to add them to this book, and you confirm their ownership and consent to our use without any further conditions.

Aloe Vera

A succulent plant known for its thick, fleshy leaves filled with a gel-like substance. It has been used for centuries in traditional medicine for its healing properties. Aloe Vera is rich in vitamins, minerals, enzymes, and amino acids. It's primarily used for skin care, aiding in the healing of burns, cuts, and other skin irritations.

Digestive System

Stomach and Intestines: Aloe Vera aids in digestion, soothes stomach lining, and can relieve constipation. It acts as a natural laxative and helps maintain healthy intestinal flora.

Immune System

Overall Function: Boosts the immune system with its anti-inflammatory and antimicrobial properties, helping to fight infections and heal wounds.

Skin and Integumentary System

Skin: Beneficial for hydrating skin, healing burns, reducing acne, and treating other skin conditions. Also helps in cell regeneration and has anti-aging properties!

How to Grow Aloe Vera

- **Selecting the Right Variety:** Aloe Barbadensis Miller is the most beneficial for medicinal purposes. Starting with offshoots or "starts" from an established plant is preferable as it ensures faster growth and success. These are readily available in nurseries, garden centers, or online plant stores.

- **Best Time to Plant Outdoors:** Spring to early summer is ideal, allowing the plant to establish before colder weather.

- **Spacing Outdoor Plants:** Plant at least 18-24 inches apart to ensure adequate space for growth and airflow.

- **Container and Soil:** Use well-draining soil, such as a cactus mix, in a pot with drainage holes to prevent waterlogging.

- **Sunlight and Location:** Aloe Vera requires about 6-8 hours of sunlight daily. In extremely hot climates, partial shade is beneficial. For indoor growth, use LED grow lights or full-spectrum bulbs.

- **Watering:** Water deeply but infrequently, allowing the soil to dry out between watering sessions.

- **Feeding:** Use a balanced, water-soluble fertilizer quarterly during the growing season.

- **Pruning and Maintenance:** Remove dead or damaged leaves at their base to encourage new growth and maintain plant health.

- **Pest and Disease Management:** Monitor for common issues like scale insects and fungal rot; treat with organic pesticides and ensure good air circulation.

- **Overwintering:** In cold climates, move outdoor plants indoors to provide protection from frost.

- **Propagation:** Easily propagated from offsets or leaf cuttings in spring or summer.
- **Harvesting:** Leaves can be harvested as needed by cutting close to the base, ensuring sustainable plant growth.
- **Climate Considerations:** Best grown in warm, arid climates but adaptable to indoor environments with controlled conditions.

How to Use Aloe Vera

Salves-Topical Applications: Aloe vera gel is extracted from the leaf and used in creams, ointments, and poultices for its soothing and healing properties. Apply directly to the skin to treat burns, wounds, and skin irritations.

Compresses: Aloe vera gel or juice can be used to soak a clean cloth, creating a compress that can be applied to affected areas to reduce inflammation and soothe pain.

Juices: The gel from aloe vera leaves is commonly consumed as a juice. It is well known for its digestive benefits and can be taken internally to support gastrointestinal health and boost your immune system.

Culinary Uses: While not common, aloe vera gel can be used in small amounts in culinary preparations, such as smoothies and desserts, for its health benefits.

Ease to Grow: 2 - 3 Low Maintenance

Aloe Vera is easy to grow and maintain. It prefers well-draining soil, requires infrequent watering, and thrives in warm, sunny conditions. It's a hardy plant that doesn't need much attention and is perfect for beginners in gardening.

Angelica

Known for its sweetly scented umbels and robust stature, a revered plant in the herbal world. Its towering presence in the garden mirrors its significant impact on human health, particularly within traditional medicine systems. Angelica is primarily associated with the digestive and respiratory systems, offering soothing and stimulating properties.

Digestive System

Stomach: Angelica stimulates appetite, improves digestion, and alleviates stomach discomfort.

Intestines: It helps relieve intestinal gas, bloating, and spasms, promoting gut health.

Liver: Also supports liver function, aiding in detoxification processes.

Respiratory System

Lungs: Acts as an expectorant, clearing mucus from the respiratory tract.

Throat: Soothes sore throats and reduces inflammation.

Nasal passages: Relieves congestion and facilitates easier breathing.

How to Grow Angelica

- **Selecting the Right Variety:** Angelica Archangelica is the most common medicinal variety. It's best to start with seedlings or division of roots, as seeds can be difficult to germinate. Purchase from reputable nurseries or online herb specialists.

- **Best Time to Plant Outdoors:** Early spring or autumn, as Angelica prefers cooler temperatures to begin its growth cycle.
- **Spacing Outdoor Plants:** Plant seedlings or root divisions about 2 to 3 feet apart to accommodate their wide spread.
- **Container Use and Soil:** Use large containers with well-draining soil rich in organic matter; angelica thrives in moist, fertile earth.
- **Sunlight and Location:** Prefers partial shade; too much sun can scorch leaves. In artificial settings, use grow lights mimicking natural light cycles.
- **Watering:** Keep soil consistently moist but not waterlogged; angelica does not tolerate drought.
- **Feeding:** Enrich soil with compost or a balanced organic fertilizer in spring and mid-summer.
- **Pruning and Maintenance:** Snip off dead flowers to promote growth and prevent self-seeding.
- **Pest and Disease Management:** Watch for aphids and treat with natural insecticides; prevent root rot by ensuring good drainage.
- **Overwintering:** In colder climates, mulch around the base to protect roots from freezing.
- **Propagation:** Best propagated by root division in autumn.
- **Harvesting:** Leaves and stems in spring, roots in autumn after the first year of growth.
- **Climate Considerations:** Angelica thrives in cool, temperate climates with consistent moisture, not suited for extreme heat or dry conditions.

How to Use Angelica

Herbal Teas or Infusions: Soak dried or fresh Angelica leaves or roots in hot water to create a soothing tea that aids digestion and relieves respiratory conditions.

Tinctures: The roots or seeds of Angelica are soaked in alcohol to extract their active compounds, creating a tincture that can help with digestive issues and nerve pain.

Salves-Topical Applications: The extracted oil from Angelica seeds or roots is mixed with a carrier oil and beeswax to make salves or ointments for skin ailments and joint pain.

Compresses: Soaked Angelica leaves, or a decoction of the roots, can be applied as a compress to relieve pain or inflammation in muscles and joints.

Aromatherapy & Essential Oils: Essential oil derived from Angelica can be used in diffusers or applied topically when diluted with a carrier oil to help reduce anxiety and promote relaxation.

Herbal Baths: Adding Angelica leaves or a decoction of the roots to bath water can help soothe skin irritations and promote relaxation.

Steam Inhalation: Inhaling the steam from a decoction of Angelica can relieve respiratory conditions like colds and coughs.

Decoctions: Simmering Angelica roots or seeds creates a strong decoction that can be taken internally to help with digestive issues and respiratory health.

Syrups: A syrup made from the root of Angelica can soothe coughs and sore throats.

Gargles & Mouthwashes: A mild decoction of Angelica can be used as a gargle or mouthwash to treat throat irritations and oral infections.

Powders: Dried Angelica root can be ground into a powder and used in capsules or as a spice in cooking.

Juices: Juice from fresh Angelica leaves or stems can be consumed for its health benefits, particularly for digestive health.

Culinary Uses: Angelica stems and leaves can be used in cooking, particularly in sweet dishes and confections, for flavor and digestive benefits.

Ease to Grow: 3-5 - Medium Maintenance

Angelica grows well in cool, moist climates with partial shade. It requires regular watering and fertile, well-draining soil. While not overly demanding, some knowledge of herb gardening is beneficial to manage its growth cycle and harvest appropriately.

Anise

Known scientifically as Pimpinella Anisum, is a flavorful herb renowned for its fragrant seeds that taste like licorice. It's not just a culinary delight but also packed with medicinal benefits, especially for the digestive and respiratory systems.

Digestive System

Stomach: Anise aids in digestion, reducing bloating, and easing cramps by relaxing the stomach muscles.

Intestines: It can alleviate intestinal gas and discomfort, promoting a healthy digestive process.

Respiratory System

Lungs: Anise acts as an expectorant, helping to clear congestion and ease coughing.

Airways: Soothes irritation in the throat and respiratory tract, making breathing easier.

How to Grow Anise

- **Selecting the Right Variety:** Anise is typically grown from its seeds, with primarily one common variety used for both culinary and medicinal purposes. Seeds are available at garden centers or online seed stores.
- **Best Time to Plant Outdoors:** Plant anise seeds in late spring, after the last frost, to ensure the soil is warm enough for germination.
- **Spacing Outdoor Plants:** Space anise plants 12 to 18 inches apart to allow room for growth.
- **Container Use and Soil:** Anise grows well in pots with well-draining soil rich in organic matter. A pot at least 10 inches deep is suitable for root development.
- **Sunlight and Location:** Anise prefers full sun, requiring at least six hours of direct sunlight daily. If using artificial lighting, full-spectrum grow lights mimic natural sunlight well.
- **Watering:** Keep the soil moist but not waterlogged. Anise needs regular watering, especially during dry periods.
- **Feeding:** Fertilize with a balanced, all-purpose fertilizer every few weeks to support growth.
- **Pruning and Maintenance:** Regularly remove dead flowers to promote new growth and prevent the plant from becoming leggy (long, thin, weak stems)

- **Pest and Disease Management:** Watch for common pests like aphids and treat with natural pesticides. Fungal diseases can be managed by ensuring good air circulation and not overwatering.
- **Overwintering:** In colder climates, anise may not survive the winter outdoors. Consider growing in pots that can be brought indoors.
- **Propagation:** Anise can be propagated from seeds. Plant fresh seeds each year for the best yield.
- **Harvesting:** Harvest anise seeds in late summer, once they've turned brown but before they scatter from the plant.
- **Climate Considerations:** Anise thrives in warm, sunny climates but can grow in temperate zones with the right care. It prefers a consistent temperature without extreme changes.

How to Use Anise

Herbal Teas or Infusions: Anise seeds are soaked in hot water to create a tea that aids in digestion and relieves flatulence.

Tinctures: Anise seed tincture is used for its digestive and expectorant properties, helping with coughs and bronchial issues.

Decoctions: A strong decoction made from anise seeds can relieve colic and cramps.

Syrups: Anise syrup is often used to treat coughs and sore throats due to its soothing properties.

Gargles & Mouthwashes: Aniseed-infused water can be used as a gargle or mouthwash to freshen breath and promote oral health.

Powders: Anise seeds are ground into powder for culinary uses and as a digestive aid.

Culinary Uses: Anise seeds are widely used in cooking and baking for their distinctive licorice-like flavor and digestive benefits.

Ease to Grow: 2-4, Low Maintenance

Anise is relatively easy to grow, requiring well-drained soil and a sunny location. It can be grown from seed and tends to thrive with minimal care, making it suitable for novice gardeners. Regular watering and occasional feeding will yield a healthy anise plant with aromatic seeds.

Ashwagandha

Also known as Withania Somnifera, is a renowned herb in Ayurvedic medicine, celebrated for its properties that help the body manage stress. It boosts energy, improves concentration, and can alleviate anxiety and depression. This herb strengthens the immune system, enhances stamina, and has been shown to improve sexual health by increasing libido and combating erectile dysfunction.

Nervous System

Stress and Anxiety: Ashwagandha reduces cortisol levels, alleviating stress and reducing anxiety symptoms.

Endocrine System

Thyroid Function: Can normalize thyroid hormone levels, particularly in hypothyroidism, by stimulating thyroid activity.

Immune System

Immune Support: Boosts the immune system by increasing the production of white blood cells, enhancing the body's resistance to illness.

Reproductive System

Fertility and Libido: Ashwagandha supports reproductive health by enhancing libido and increasing sperm count and motility in men, and improving hormonal balance in women.

How to Grow Ashwagandha

- **Selecting the Right Variety:** Ashwagandha prefers warm climates but can be grown in temperate zones. Start with seeds or small plants from reputable nurseries or online stores.
- **Best Time to Plant Outdoors:** Plant in spring after the last frost to ensure optimal growth.
- **Spacing Outdoor Plants:** Space plants about 18 inches apart to allow for adequate growth and airflow.
- **Container Use and Soil:** Use well-draining soil in containers or raised beds to prevent root rot.
- **Sunlight and Location:** Requires full sun, around 6-8 hours daily; can use grow lights for indoor cultivation.
- **Watering:** Water regularly but allow the soil to dry between waterings to prevent overwatering.
- **Feeding:** Apply a balanced, slow-release fertilizer at the beginning of the growing season.
- **Pruning and Maintenance:** Remove dead or yellowing leaves to promote healthy growth.
- **Pest and Disease Management:** Monitor for common pests like aphids; use organic pesticides if necessary.

- **Overwintering:** In cooler climates, mulch around the base to protect roots from freezing.
- **Propagation:** Propagate from seeds or cuttings in early spring.
- **Harvesting:** Roots are typically harvested in the fall of the second year; dry them properly for medicinal use.
- **Climate Considerations:** Thrives in warm to temperate climates; less successful in very cold or wet regions.

How to Use Ashwagandha

Herbal Teas or Infusions: Ashwagandha root is soaked in hot water to make a tea known for its stress-reducing and rejuvenating properties.

Tinctures: The roots are often used to prepare tinctures that help in regulating stress hormones and improving overall vitality.

Salves-Topical Applications: Ashwagandha-infused oils can be turned into salves or ointments, applied topically to reduce joint inflammation and skin irritations.

Compresses: A compress soaked in ashwagandha tea can be applied to areas of swelling or muscle pain for relief.

Decoctions: The roots can be boiled to make a strong decoction, consumed to enhance stamina and energy levels.

Powders: Ashwagandha root is dried and powdered, commonly used as a dietary supplement for its adaptogenic effects (helps the body adapt and cope with stress).

Juices: Though less common, the fresh roots can be juiced and taken for its therapeutic benefits.

Culinary Uses: The powdered form of ashwagandha is sometimes used in small amounts in traditional Indian dishes for its health benefits.

Ease to Grow: 3-5, Medium Maintenance

Ashwagandha is a hardy plant that can grow in arid conditions and requires minimal water once established. It prefers warm climates and well-drained soil. While it's not very demanding, some attention to soil quality and watering can enhance the growth and potency of the roots, which are the most commonly used part of the plant for medicinal purposes.

Astragalus

Also known as Astragalus Membranaceus, a traditional Chinese medicinal herb used for centuries to boost the immune system and combat stress. Its roots contain compounds that enhance the body's natural defense mechanisms and promote overall vitality. Astragalus is particularly beneficial for:

Immune System

White Blood Cell Stimulation: Astragalus enhances immune function by stimulating white blood cell production, bolstering the body's defense mechanisms.

Cardiovascular System

Heart Function: It is known to improve heart function and increase blood flow, essential for cardiovascular health.

Respiratory System

Lung Protection: Astragalus supports lung health by acting as a protective barrier against respiratory infections and stressors.

Endocrine System

Hormonal Balance: Astragalus helps to regulate hormones, contributing to the stability of the body's endocrine functions.

Gastrointestinal System

Intestinal Health: By promoting the repair of intestinal mucosa, Astragalus enhances nutrient absorption and maintains digestive tract health.

How to Grow Astragalus

- **Selecting the Right Variety:** Astragalus Membranaceus is the most commonly used variety for medicinal purposes. It's preferable to start with seeds or root cuttings, available from specialized online herb nurseries or local garden centers. Research suppliers for quality and authenticity.
- **Best Time to Plant Outdoors:** Plant in early spring after the last frost. Seeds germinate better with cold beginnings, so consider sowing them in fall if your climate allows.
- **Spacing Outdoor Plants:** Space plants or seeds about 18 to 24 inches apart to allow room for growth.
- **Container Use and Soil:** Astragalus thrives in well-draining, sandy loam soil with a neutral to slightly alkaline pH. In containers, use a mix of garden soil, sand, and compost.

- **Sunlight and Location:** Prefers full sun, needing at least 6 to 8 hours of direct sunlight daily. Can tolerate partial shade but may affect root development.
- **Watering:** Water regularly to keep the soil moist but not waterlogged. Reduce watering during the winter dormancy period.
- **Feeding:** Apply a balanced, slow-release fertilizer in early spring to support growth.
- **Pruning and Maintenance:** Minimal pruning is needed. Remove any dead or yellowing leaves to maintain plant health.
- **Pest and Disease Management:** Watch for common pests like aphids and treat with organic pesticides. Root rot can occur in poorly draining soils, so ensure good soil aeration.
- **Overwintering:** In colder regions, mulch around the base to protect roots from freezing temperatures.
- **Propagation:** Propagate by dividing the roots in autumn or by sowing seeds.
- **Harvesting:** The roots are harvested in the fall of the fourth year. Dig up the roots, clean them, and dry them for medicinal use.
- **Climate Considerations:** Best grown in temperate climates. It can tolerate winter cold but not extreme heat or drought. In very cold regions, provide winter protection.

How to Use Astragalus

Herbal Teas or Infusions: Soak dried astragalus root in hot water for several minutes to make a rejuvenating tea that supports immune function.

Tinctures: Dried astragalus root can be soaked in alcohol to create a tincture, taken in small doses to enhance immunity and energy.

Decoctions: Simmer astragalus root in water for a long time to extract deep-seated nutrients, ideal for strengthening the body's defenses.

Powders: The dried root can be ground into a powder and mixed into foods or smoothies for an immune-boosting supplement.

Culinary Uses: The root can be added to soups and stews, imparting a sweet, slightly earthy flavor while boosting the dish's nutritional value.

Ease to Grow 3-4 Low to Medium Maintenance

Astragalus is generally considered a 3-4 on the scale of 1-10, making it low to medium maintenance. It is hardy and adapts well to various climates, preferring full sun and well-draining soil. With minimal pest issues and straightforward care requirements, astragalus is a good choice for gardeners looking to grow medicinal herbs.

Basil

Renowned for its aromatic leaves and robust flavor, often used in culinary dishes. Beyond its culinary appeal, basil has numerous health benefits, particularly affecting the digestive, nervous, and cardiovascular systems. It has anti-inflammatory and antibacterial properties that can enhance overall health.

Digestive System

Stomach: Basil can alleviate stomach cramps and facilitate digestion, reducing discomfort and enhancing nutrient absorption.

Nervous System

Stress Response: Basil's adaptogenic properties (meaning - helps the body adapt and cope with stress) help in managing stress and improving mental clarity.

Respiratory System

Airways: Basil acts as an expectorant, helping to clear mucus and ease breathing.

Cardiovascular System

Blood Vessels: Basil contains antioxidants that help in maintaining healthy blood vessels and reducing the risk of atherosclerosis. Its antioxidant properties protect against vascular damage and support overall cardiovascular function.

Immune System

General Immunity: The antimicrobial properties of basil boost the immune system's ability to fight off pathogens.

Skin and Integumentary System

Skin Health: Basil's antibacterial and anti-inflammatory qualities contribute to healthier skin by reducing inflammation and infections. Topically, basil can treat skin infections, improve acne, and promote wound healing due to its antibacterial and anti-inflammatory properties.

How to Grow Basil

- **Selecting the Right Variety:** Basil comes in several varieties, with Sweet Basil being the most common for culinary use. Other varieties like Thai Basil or Lemon Basil offer different flavors. Seeds or starter plants are available at garden centers or online.

- **Best Time to Plant Outdoors:** Plant basil outdoors in late spring or early summer, after the last frost.

- **Spacing Outdoor Plants:** Space plants about 12 to 18 inches apart to allow for adequate airflow and growth.

- **Container Use and Soil:** Basil thrives in well-draining soil with a neutral pH. Containers should have drainage holes to prevent waterlogging.

- **Sunlight and Location:** Basil needs 6 to 8 hours of direct sunlight daily. For artificial lighting, use full-spectrum grow lights positioned about 12 inches above the plants.

- **Watering:** Keep the soil consistently moist but not waterlogged. Water when the top inch of soil feels dry.

- **Feeding:** Use a balanced, water-soluble fertilizer every 4 to 6 weeks during the growing season.

- **Pruning and Maintenance:** Regularly snip off the tips of the branches to encourage bushier growth. Remove any dead flowers to promote more leaves.

- **Pest and Disease Management:** Watch for common pests like aphids and treat with organic insecticidal soap. Prevent fungal diseases by ensuring good air circulation and not overwatering.

- **Overwintering:** In colder climates, bring potted basil indoors or treat it as an annual and replant each year.

- **Propagation:** Propagate basil by seeds or cuttings. Place stem cuttings in water until they root, then transplant.

- **Harvesting:** Harvest leaves as needed, preferably in the morning when the oil content is highest. Use fresh, or dry and store for later use.
- **Climate Considerations:** Basil grows best in warm climates with plenty of sunlight. It can thrive in temperate zones but requires protection from frost and extreme cold.

How to Use Basil

Herbal Teas or Infusions: Soak dried basil leaves in hot water to create a soothing tea that can aid digestion and reduce stress.

Tinctures: Basil leaves are steeped in alcohol to create tinctures that can be used to improve digestion and alleviate stress.

Salves-Topical Applications: Crushed basil leaves are mixed with oils or beeswax to make creams or ointments for skin irritations and insect bites.

Compresses: Apply a cloth soaked in basil-infused water to areas of swelling or pain for relief.

Aromatherapy & Essential Oils: Basil essential oil is used in diffusers or applied topically when diluted to uplift mood and alleviate respiratory issues.

Herbal Baths: Adding basil leaves to bathwater can create a relaxing and aromatic experience that soothes the skin.

Steam Inhalation: Inhaling steam infused with basil leaves can clear nasal passages and relieve respiratory discomfort.

Decoctions: Boiling basil leaves to concentrate their oils and compounds can be used for digestive issues and as a health tonic.

Syrups: Basil can be simmered with sugar and water to create a syrup that soothes sore throats and coughs.

Gargles & Mouthwashes: A basil infusion can be used as a gargle or mouthwash to freshen breath and relieve mouth sores.

Powders: Dried and ground basil leaves can be used as a spice or for encapsulation as a dietary supplement.

Juices: Fresh basil leaves can be juiced and consumed for their health benefits.

Culinary Uses: Basil is widely used in cooking for its flavor, particularly in Italian cuisine, and offers antioxidant benefits.

Ease to Grow: 2-4, Low Maintenance

Basil is one of the easiest herbs to grow, requiring minimal care. It thrives in warm, sunny conditions and needs regular watering but well-drained soil. Basil can be grown in pots or directly in the garden, making it accessible for both outdoor and indoor environments. Its aromatic leaves not only enhance culinary dishes but also benefit health, making it a versatile and valuable plant in any herbal garden.

Bay Leaf

Known scientifically as Laurus Nobilis, is a fragrant leaf from the laurel tree, used both as a culinary herb and in traditional medicine. Rich in essential oils, vitamins, and minerals, bay leaf offers numerous health benefits. It is particularly noted for its positive effects on the digestive and respiratory systems.

Digestive System

Stomach: Bay leaf aids in digestion, stimulating gastric juice production and reducing symptoms of bloating and gas.

Intestines: It helps to regulate intestinal movements, alleviating common digestive disorders like constipation.

Respiratory System

Lungs: The compounds in bay leaf have expectorant properties, helping to loosen phlegm and relieve chest congestion.

How to Grow Bay Leaf

- **Selecting the Right Variety:** Bay Leaf trees, Laurus Nobilis, are the most common for culinary and medicinal use. Opt for nursery-grown starts as they are easier to establish than seeds. You can purchase them from garden centers or online nurseries.
- **Best Time to Plant Outdoors:** Plant in spring or autumn when the weather is mild.
- **Spacing Outdoor Plants:** Space plants 20 to 30 feet apart to allow for mature growth.
- **Container Use and Soil:** Use large containers with well-draining soil, rich in organic matter.
- **Sunlight and Location:** Bay trees thrive in full sun to partial shade. They need at least 6 hours of direct sunlight daily. If using artificial lighting, ensure it mimics the natural sunlight spectrum.
- **Watering:** Water regularly to keep the soil moist but not waterlogged.
- **Feeding:** Apply a balanced fertilizer every few months to support growth.

- **Pruning and Maintenance:** Prune to shape the tree and remove any dead or diseased leaves.
- **Pest and Disease Management:** Watch for bay leaf eaters and scale insects. Treat infestations with horticultural oils or insecticidal soaps.
- **Overwintering:** In colder zones, protect outdoor plants with mulch or move containers indoors.
- **Propagation:** Propagate by cuttings or layering in early spring or late summer.
- **Harvesting:** Harvest leaves any time, but they are most aromatic before flowering. Leaves can be used fresh or dried for later use.
- **Climate Considerations:** Bay trees are best suited to mild, wet winters and hot, dry summer climates, but can adapt to various conditions if protected from extreme cold or heat.

How to Use Bay Leaf

Herbal Teas or Infusions: Bay leaves are soaked in hot water to create a flavorful tea that aids digestion and respiratory health.

Tinctures: Bay leaf tinctures are used for its antifungal and antibacterial properties, often applied to help with skin and respiratory issues.

Salves-Topical Applications: Creams or ointments made from bay leaf extract are applied to the skin to relieve pain and inflammation.

Compresses: A compress soaked in bay leaf infusion can be applied to sore areas to reduce discomfort.

Aromatherapy & Essential Oils: Bay leaf oil is used in diffusers or applied directly to the skin for relaxation and to alleviate stress.

Herbal Baths: Adding bay leaves to bathwater can provide a soothing and aromatic experience, helping to relieve muscle tension.

Steam Inhalation: Inhaling steam infused with bay leaves can clear nasal passages and improve respiratory health.

Decoctions: A bay leaf decoction is consumed for gastrointestinal health and to boost the immune system.

Syrups: Bay leaf syrup is sometimes used to soothe sore throats and coughs.

Gargles & Mouthwashes: A gargle solution made from bay leaf infusion helps in treating oral health issues.

Powders: Bay leaf powder is used in cooking and as a seasoning to enhance flavor.

Juices: Though not common, bay leaf juice can be used for its health benefits.

Culinary Uses: Bay leaves are commonly used in cooking to flavor soups, stews, and meat dishes; they are removed before consumption.

Ease to Grow: 3-5, Low to Medium Maintenance

Bay leaf plants are fairly easy to grow, requiring well-drained soil and full sun to partial shade. They can adapt to different environments and are relatively drought-resistant once established. Regular pruning helps to maintain their shape and encourage growth. Bay leaf plants are ideal for beginners looking to add aromatic and culinary herbs to their garden.

Bee Balm

Also known as Monarda, is a fragrant herb renowned for its ornamental and medicinal properties. Its vibrant flowers and aromatic leaves are not only a magnet for bees and butterflies but also hold significant therapeutic benefits. Traditionally, Bee Balm has been used to alleviate digestive issues, soothe respiratory conditions, and treat skin ailments due to its antiseptic and anti-inflammatory properties.

Respiratory System

Lungs: Bee Balm helps in alleviating respiratory conditions, acting as an expectorant to clear mucus.

Throat: Soothes sore throats and reduces coughing, providing relief from irritation.

Digestive System

Stomach: Bee Balm can ease stomach pain and support digestion, helping to relieve gastric discomfort.

Intestines: Assists in reducing intestinal bloating and gas, enhancing overall digestive health.

Immune System

Overall Immunity: Bee Balm's antimicrobial properties strengthen the immune response and help fight infections.

Skin and Integumentary System

Skin: Its antiseptic properties make it useful for treating skin infections and wounds, promoting healing and reducing inflammation.

How to Grow Bee Balm

- **Selecting the Right Variety:** Bee Balm has several varieties, each with unique characteristics. Look for varieties like 'Jacob

112

Cline' for its robust growth and mildew resistance, 'Marshall's Delight' for pink flowers and disease resistance, or 'Pardon My Purple' for compact growth. Seeds, plant starts, or cuttings are suitable for propagation. Preferred methods may depend on the variety and your gardening setup. You can purchase these from nurseries, garden centers, or online retailers specializing in herb plants.

- **Best Time to Plant Outdoors:** The ideal time to plant Bee Balm outdoors is in the spring after the last frost or in the early fall to allow roots to establish before winter.
- **Spacing Outdoor Plants:** Space Bee Balm plants about 18 to 24 inches apart to ensure adequate air circulation and reduce the risk of powdery mildew.
- **Container Use and Soil:** Bee Balm thrives in well-draining soil with a pH between 6.0 and 7.0. For container planting, use a pot with drainage holes and a standard potting mix with added compost.
- **Sunlight and Location:** Bee Balm prefers full sun, requiring at least 6 hours of direct sunlight daily. In hot climates, partial afternoon shade can prevent overheating. For artificial lighting, use full-spectrum grow lights positioned 12-16 inches above the plants.
- **Watering:** Keep the soil consistently moist but not waterlogged. Water at the base of the plant to avoid wetting the foliage, which can lead to disease.
- **Feeding:** Fertilize Bee Balm in the spring with a balanced, slow-release fertilizer to support growth and blooming.
- **Pruning and Maintenance:** Regularly snip off old blooms to encourage more flowers. Prune back in late fall or early spring to maintain shape and promote healthy growth.
- **Pest and Disease Management:** Watch for signs of powdery mildew, rust, or aphid infestations. Treat diseases

with fungicides and manage pests with insecticidal soap or neem oil as needed.

- **Overwintering:** In colder zones, mulch around the base of the plant to protect roots from freezing. In milder climates, Bee Balm may remain evergreen or semi-evergreen.
- **Propagation:** Propagate Bee Balm by division in the spring or autumn. Cuttings can also be rooted in water or soil.
- **Harvesting:** Harvest leaves and flowers in the morning after dew has evaporated. Use fresh or dry them for later use. Bee Balm is known for its aromatic leaves and flowers, which can be used to make tea or as a culinary herb.
- **Climate Considerations:** Bee Balm prefers temperate climates and needs protection from extreme cold and excessive heat. Optimal growth is achieved in areas with distinct seasons and moderate temperatures.

How to Use Bee Balm

Herbal Teas or Infusions: Soak the leaves or flowers in hot water to make a tea that helps with digestive and respiratory issues. The aroma and compounds in the tea can also reduce stress and promote relaxation.

Tinctures: Bee Balm leaves and flowers can be soaked in alcohol to create a tincture, which can be used for its antiseptic properties and to help with digestive problems.

Salves-Topical Applications: The plant's leaves, when infused in a carrier oil, can be used in creams and ointments to treat skin irritations, minor wounds, and burns.

Compresses: A cloth soaked in Bee Balm tea can be applied to the skin to relieve pain and inflammation, especially in cases of insect bites or rashes.

Aromatherapy & Essential Oils: Essential oil derived from Bee

Balm can be used in aromatherapy for its soothing properties, helping to alleviate stress and insomnia.

Herbal Baths: Adding Bee Balm to bathwater can create a therapeutic herbal bath, soothing skin irritations and promoting relaxation.

Steam Inhalation: Inhaling the steam from boiled Bee Balm leaves can relieve nasal congestion and respiratory issues.

Decoctions: A strong Bee Balm decoction can be used for gargling to soothe sore throats or as a digestive aid when consumed.

Syrups: Bee Balm syrup, made by reducing a decoction with sugar, can soothe coughs and sore throats.

Gargles & Mouthwashes: A Bee Balm infusion can be used as a gargle or mouthwash to treat oral infections and sore throats.

Powders: Dried Bee Balm can be ground into a powder and used for culinary purposes or as a natural remedy.

Juices: The juice extracted from Bee Balm leaves can be used medicinally for its antiseptic and antibacterial properties.

Culinary Uses: Bee Balm leaves can be used fresh or dried to flavor foods, offering a mint-like taste and digestive benefits.

Ease to Grow: 3-5, Low to Medium Maintenance

Bee Balm is relatively easy to grow, requiring minimal care once established. It prefers well-drained soil with a good amount of sunlight but can tolerate partial shade. The plant is drought-tolerant but benefits from occasional watering during prolonged dry spells. Pruning dead flowers can promote more blooms. Bee Balm attracts pollinators, enhancing garden biodiversity.

Bergamot

Scientifically known as Monarda, is renowned for its distinct citrus aroma and medicinal properties. It is particularly prized in treating digestive and respiratory issues, thanks to its antiseptic and anti-inflammatory properties. Bergamot's uplifting scent also makes it a popular choice in aromatherapy, providing nervous system support by alleviating stress and anxiety.

Digestive System

Stomach: Bergamot oil stimulates digestion, easing discomfort like bloating and cramps.

Intestines: Its antibacterial qualities can help balance intestinal flora and reduce infections.

Respiratory System

Lungs: The plant acts as an expectorant, aiding in loosening phlegm and relieving congestion.

Bronchi: Its anti-inflammatory effects help soothe bronchial irritation.

Nervous System

Brain: The soothing aroma of bergamot oil helps reduce stress and anxiety, promoting mental well-being.

Nerves: It has a calming effect, aiding in relaxation and potentially alleviating symptoms of depression.

Skin and Integumentary System

Skin: Bergamot's antiseptic properties make it beneficial for treating skin infections and enhancing skin health.

Immune System

Overall Immunity: The antimicrobial properties of bergamot can help strengthen the body's defense against infections.

How to Grow Bergamot

- **Selecting the Right Variety:** Choose varieties like Monarda Didyma or Monarda Fistulosa for their robust flavor and medicinal properties. Purchase seeds or starts from reputable nurseries or online stores specializing in medicinal herbs.
- **Best Time to Plant Outdoors:** Plant in early spring after the last frost, or in autumn in warmer climates, to allow roots to establish before the hot or cold season.
- **Spacing Outdoor Plants:** Space plants 18 to 24 inches apart to ensure adequate air circulation and reduce the risk of fungal diseases.
- **Container Use and Soil:** Use large pots with drainage holes, filled with well-draining soil rich in organic matter; a pH of 6.0 to 7.0 is ideal for optimal growth.
- **Sunlight and Location:** Requires full sun to partial shade, about 6 to 8 hours of direct sunlight daily. If using artificial

lighting, opt for full-spectrum LED grow lights positioned 12-24 inches above plants.

- **Watering:** Keep the soil consistently moist but not waterlogged; water at the base of the plant to prevent leaf diseases.
- **Feeding:** Fertilize monthly with a balanced organic fertilizer to promote healthy growth and flower production.
- **Pruning and Maintenance:** Regularly snip off dead flowers to encourage more blooms and prevent self-seeding. Trim back in late fall or early spring to promote bushier growth.
- **Pest and Disease Management:** Monitor for common pests like aphids and spider mites. Treat fungal diseases like powdery mildew with organic fungicides and ensure good air circulation.
- **Overwintering:** In colder zones, mulch around the base to protect roots from freezing. In milder climates, cut back foliage to ground level in late autumn.
- **Propagation:** Propagate by seed in spring or by division in spring or autumn. Root cuttings can also be taken in winter for new plants.
- **Harvesting:** Harvest leaves and flowers in the morning after dew has dried for the highest essential oil concentration. Leaves can be used fresh or dried for later use.
- **Climate Considerations:** Thrives in temperate climates but can tolerate various conditions if well-managed. Avoid waterlogged soils and extremely hot or frost-prone areas.

How to Use Bergamot

Herbal Teas or Infusions: Soak dried bergamot leaves or flowers in hot water to create a soothing tea that aids digestion and relieves stress.

Tinctures: Bergamot leaves or flowers are steeped in alcohol to make a tincture, which can be used to alleviate digestive issues and promote relaxation.

Salves-Topical Applications: The oil extracted from bergamot is used in creams or ointments to treat skin conditions like eczema and acne due to its antibacterial properties.

Compresses: A cloth soaked in bergamot infusion can be applied to the skin to relieve pain and inflammation, especially in cases of minor burns or insect bites.

Aromatherapy & Essential Oils: Bergamot oil is used in diffusers or can be applied topically (diluted) to uplift mood, reduce stress, and improve sleep quality.

Herbal Baths: Adding bergamot leaves or oil to bathwater can create a relaxing and fragrant experience, helping to soothe skin irritations and relieve stress.

Steam Inhalation: Inhaling steam infused with bergamot oil can alleviate respiratory issues, clear nasal passages, and promote a sense of relaxation.

Decoctions: A strong brew made from simmering bergamot plant parts, particularly beneficial for respiratory health and as a digestive aid.

Syrups: Bergamot infused syrup can soothe sore throats and coughs when used as a medicinal remedy.

Gargles & Mouthwashes: A bergamot infusion can be used as a gargle or mouthwash to freshen breath and kill bacteria.

Powders: Dried bergamot leaves ground into a powder can be used in culinary creations or as a natural fragrance.

Juices: Fresh bergamot leaves and flowers can be juiced and consumed for their health benefits.

Culinary Uses: Fresh or dried bergamot leaves are used to flavor dishes, imparting a unique citrus-like taste to salads, sauces, and teas.

Bergamot is a hardy perennial that thrives with minimal care, making it suitable for beginner gardeners. It prefers well-drained soil, moderate watering, and full sun to partial shade. Regular pruning and snipping off of dead flowers encourage growth and prevent overcrowding.

Burdock

A biennial plant known for its burr-seed heads and deep roots. It has been traditionally used for purifying blood, promoting skin health, and supporting the digestive system. Its roots, rich in inulin (a dietary fiber), can help regulate blood sugar and improve gut flora. Burdock's antioxidant properties also aid in liver detoxification and overall immune support.

Digestive System

Stomach: Burdock aids in digestion by increasing stomach acid secretion, improving appetite, and nutrient absorption.

Intestines: It acts as a prebiotic, nourishing beneficial gut bacteria, and promoting bowel regularity.

Skin and Integumentary System

Skin: Burdock root's anti-inflammatory and antibacterial properties help treat skin conditions like acne, eczema, and psoriasis.

Lymphatic System

Lymph nodes: It enhances lymphatic drainage, helping to detoxify the body and improve immune function.

Endocrine System

Pancreas: Burdock can help regulate blood sugar levels, benefiting those with diabetes.

How to Grow Burdock

- **Selecting the Right Variety:** Choose Arctium Lappa or Arctium Minus for medicinal use; both are known for their robust root systems. Starting from seeds is common, but young plants or root cuttings can also be used. Seeds are available online or at specialty garden stores.
- **Best Time to Plant Outdoors:** Plant seeds in late fall or early spring, as they need cold to germinate. For root cuttings, plant in early spring.
- **Spacing Outdoor Plants:** Space plants about 24-36 inches apart, as burdock needs room to grow its large leaves and deep roots.
- **Container Use and Soil:** Large containers with well-draining soil rich in organic matter are ideal. Burdock prefers a slightly sandy soil for better root development.
- **Sunlight and Location:** Requires full sun to partial shade, with at least 6 hours of direct sunlight daily. Can use grow lights for indoor growth, placed 24-30 inches above the plants.

- **Watering:** Water regularly to keep the soil moist but not waterlogged. Deep watering encourages root growth.
- **Feeding:** Apply a balanced organic fertilizer in the growing season to support leaf and root development.
- **Pruning and Maintenance:** Remove dead flowers to prevent self-seeding and manage plant spread. Regularly check and remove any wilted or damaged leaves.
- **Pest and Disease Management:** Watch for aphids and leaf spot. Use organic pesticides and ensure good air circulation to prevent fungal diseases.
- **Overwintering:** In colder zones, mulch around the plants to protect the roots from freezing.
- **Propagation:** Can be propagated by seed or division of root cuttings in early spring.
- **Harvesting:** Harvest roots in late fall of the first year or early spring of the second year. Leaves can be picked when young and tender.
- **Climate Considerations:** Thrives in temperate climates, but prefers regions with cold winters for seed stratification (or initial development).

How to Use Burdock

Herbal Teas or Infusions: Soak burdock root in hot water to create a detoxifying tea that aids digestion and purifies the blood.

Tinctures: Burdock root tincture is used for its blood-purifying and liver-detoxifying effects, taken in small doses.

Salves-Topical Applications: Crushed burdock leaves or root extract is used in ointments to soothe skin conditions like eczema and acne.

Decoctions: A strong burdock root decoction can be consumed to improve overall digestion and support skin health.

Powders: Dried and powdered burdock root is added to health supplements for its detoxifying properties.

Culinary Uses: Young burdock roots are edible and can be used in soups, stews, and stir-fries, known for their earthy, sweet flavor and crunchy texture.

Ease to Grow: 3-5, Low Maintenance

Burdock is a hardy plant that adapts well to various soil types and conditions. It requires minimal care once established, thriving in both full sun and partial shade. Regular watering and basic weed control are sufficient to ensure a good yield of roots and leaves.

Calendula

Commonly known as marigold, is renowned for its vibrant yellow and orange flowers that offer not just aesthetic pleasure but also a multitude of medicinal properties. This plant is particularly celebrated for its healing effects on the skin, making it a staple in herbal remedies for cuts, burns, and bruises due to its anti-inflammatory and antimicrobial attributes.

Skin and Integumentary System

Epidermis: Calendula soothes irritated skin, reduces redness, and accelerates wound healing.

Dermis: Enhances collagen production, aiding in the repair of skin tissue.

Sweat glands: With its antifungal properties, calendula helps in treating skin infections.

Immune System

Lymph nodes: Stimulates lymphatic drainage, which enhances immune response and reduces swelling.

White blood cells: Boosts the activity of white blood cells, aiding in the body's defense against pathogens.

Digestive System

Stomach: Calendula tea is used to heal gastric ulcers and relieve indigestion.

Intestines: Its anti-inflammatory properties help soothe inflamed intestinal linings.

How to Grow Calendula

- **Selecting the Right Variety:** Calendula comes in various types; the most common are Calendula Officinalis varieties known for their medicinal properties. It's often best to start with seeds or seedlings, available at nurseries or online. Choose a variety that suits your climate and soil conditions.

- **Best Time to Plant Outdoors:** Plant calendula in early spring after the risk of frost has passed. In warmer climates, it can also be planted in the autumn for winter blooms.

- **Spacing Outdoor Plants:** Space plants about 8 to 12 inches apart to allow for ample air circulation and sunlight, reducing the risk of fungal diseases.

- **Container Use and Soil:** Calendula thrives in well-draining soil with a neutral to slightly acidic pH. In containers, use a high-quality potting mix to ensure good drainage.
- **Sunlight and Location:** Prefers full sun but can tolerate partial shade. Aim for at least 6 hours of direct sunlight daily. If using artificial lighting, LED grow lights are effective; place them about 12 inches above the plants.
- **Watering:** Keep the soil evenly moist but not waterlogged. Water at the base of the plant to avoid wetting the foliage, which can lead to disease.
- **Feeding:** Calendula is not a heavy feeder, but a balanced, slow-release fertilizer at planting time can enhance growth and flowering.
- **Pruning and Maintenance:** Regularly removing dead flowers encourages more flowering, to maintain plant health and appearance.
- **Pest and Disease Management:** Watch for common pests like aphids and slugs. Treat with organic pesticides if necessary. Prevent fungal diseases by ensuring good air flow around plants.
- **Overwintering:** In colder regions, calendula may not survive freezing temperatures, so collect seeds for replanting or use mulch to protect roots in milder climates.
- **Propagation:** Easily propagated from seeds; sow directly in the ground or start indoors. Seeds typically germinate in 5 to 14 days.
- **Harvesting:** Flowers are best harvested in the morning after the dew has dried. Use them fresh or dry them for later use. Leaves and stems can also be used for their medicinal properties.
- **Climate Considerations:** Calendula grows best in temperate climates with moderate temperatures. Thriving in areas with

mild winters and warm summers.

How to Use Calendula

Herbal Teas or Infusions: Calendula flowers can be soaked in hot water to make a soothing herbal tea or infusion that supports skin health and digestion.

Tinctures: Calendula petals can be used in alcohol to create a concentrated herbal extract used for skin healing and inflammation relief.

Salves-Topical Applications: Calendula-infused creams or ointments are applied topically to promote wound healing, soothe skin irritations, and reduce inflammation.

Compresses: Calendula petals can be steeped in warm water, then applied as a compress to relieve minor skin irritations or inflammation.

Aromatherapy & Essential Oils: Calendula essential oil can be used in aromatherapy for its calming and skin-healing properties. It can also be inhaled directly or diluted for topical application.

Herbal Baths: Calendula flowers can be added to bathwater for a soothing and skin-nourishing herbal bath experience.

Steam Inhalation: Adding Calendula to a steam inhalation can help relieve respiratory congestion and soothe irritated airways.

Decoctions: Calendula petals can be simmered in water to create a strong herbal decoction used internally for digestive support or externally for skin health.

Syrups: Calendula petals can be infused in a syrup base for a sweet and medicinal syrup used to soothe sore throats or support immune health.

Gargles & Mouthwashes: Calendula-infused gargles or mouthwashes can help soothe oral irritations, promote gum health, and freshen breath.

Powders: Dried Calendula petals can be ground into a fine powder and used in various herbal preparations, such as capsules or topical applications.

Juices: Calendula flowers can be juiced for their therapeutic properties, such as supporting digestive health or providing a mild detoxification effect.

Culinary Uses: Calendula petals can be used as a colorful and nutritious addition to salads, soups, and other culinary dishes.

Ease to Grow: 3-5, Low to Medium Maintenance

Calendula is relatively easy to grow, requiring regular watering and well-drained soil. It thrives in full sun to partial shade and can tolerate cooler temperatures. Regular removal of dead flowers promotes continuous flowering. Overall, it is a rewarding herb to cultivate with moderate care.

Caraway

Known scientifically as Carum Carvi, is a biennial (2 year cycle) plant widely recognized for its culinary and medicinal uses. Its seeds are particularly valued for their distinctive flavor and health benefits. These benefits make caraway a versatile plant in both culinary and medicinal contexts, often used in the form of seeds, essential oils, or herbal teas. Its multifaceted properties align with various systems in the body, making it a valuable herb in holistic health practices.

Digestive System

Stomach: Caraway seeds can soothe the stomach, relieve indigestion, and reduce gas formation, enhancing overall digestive health.

Intestines: The seeds help in regulating bowel movements and alleviating symptoms of irritable bowel syndrome (IBS).

Respiratory System

Bronchi: Caraway's expectorant properties aid in loosening mucus, easing its expulsion and relieving coughs, improving bronchial health.

Cardiovascular System

Blood vessels: Caraway's anti-inflammatory and antioxidative components may help in maintaining healthy blood vessels, potentially reducing the risk of cardiovascular diseases.

Heart: The seeds are thought to have heart-protective qualities, possibly due to their ability to regulate cholesterol levels and enhance heart health.

How to Grow Caraway

- **Selecting the Right Variety:** Caraway comes mainly in one species, Carum Carvi. It's preferable to start with seeds, as they germinate easily. Seeds are available at garden centers or online seed stores. Look for seeds labeled as high germination rate for best results.
- **Best Time to Plant Outdoors:** Plant caraway seeds in late fall or early spring. In fall, they will germinate and overwinter as small plants, then resume growth in spring.
- **Spacing Outdoor Plants:** Sow seeds directly in the ground, spacing them 6 to 8 inches apart in rows that are 18 inches apart to allow room for growth.

- **Container Use and Soil:** Caraway thrives in well-drained soil with a pH between 6.0 and 7.5. If growing in containers, ensure they have good drainage holes and use a mix of potting soil and compost.
- **Sunlight and Location:** Caraway plants prefer full sun but can tolerate partial shade. They need around 6 to 8 hours of sunlight daily. If using artificial lighting, LED grow lights can be effective, positioned about 12 inches above the plants.
- **Watering:** Water regularly, keeping the soil moist but not waterlogged. Caraway does not tolerate drought well, so consistent watering is important.
- **Feeding:** Fertilize caraway plants with a balanced liquid fertilizer every 4 to 6 weeks during the growing season.
- **Pruning and Maintenance:** Remove dead flowers or spent blooms to encourage more growth and prevent self-seeding (if not desired).
- **Pest and Disease Management:** Monitor for common garden pests like aphids and treat with organic pesticides if necessary. Caraway is relatively disease-resistant but watch for root rot in overly wet conditions.
- **Overwintering:** In colder climates, mulch around the base of the plants to protect them through winter.
- **Propagation:** Caraway can be propagated by seeds. Allow some plants to go to seed and collect these for next season's planting.
- **Harvesting:** Harvest caraway seeds when they turn brown and the seed heads are dry, typically in late summer. Cut the seed heads and dry them before shaking out the seeds.
- **Climate Considerations:** Caraway grows best in temperate climates with well-defined seasons. It can tolerate cold winters and has a preference for cooler summer temperatures.

How to Use Caraway

Herbal Teas or Infusions: Soak caraway seeds in hot water to create a digestive aiding tea.

Tinctures: Extract caraway components in alcohol to use for digestive relief of discomfort.

Salves-Topical Applications: Incorporate caraway oil in creams or ointments for anti-inflammatory and antispasmodic skin benefits.

Compresses: Apply cloths soaked in caraway-infused water to the skin to relieve pain and inflammation.

Aromatherapy & Essential Oils: Inhale caraway essential oil or apply it topically for digestive and respiratory health.

Decoctions: Boil caraway seeds to make a strong liquid used to ease digestive issues.

Syrups: Use caraway extract in syrups for cough and sore throat relief.

Powders: Ground caraway seeds are used in cooking to aid digestion and add flavor.

Culinary Uses: Caraway seeds are widely used in cooking for their distinct flavor and digestive benefits.

Ease to Grow: 3-5, Low to Medium Maintenance

Caraway is fairly easy to grow, requiring well-drained soil and a sunny location. It's resilient to most pests and diseases, making it a good choice for beginners in gardening.

Cardamom

Often referred to as the "queen of spices,", cardamom is a perennial plant native to India and known for its aromatic seeds. Widely used in culinary applications, cardamom also boasts several health benefits.

Digestive System

Stomach: Cardamom enhances digestion, prevents stomach ulcers, and reduces nausea.

Intestines: It alleviates bloating and gas, stimulating the intestinal lining's function.

Respiratory System

Lungs: Its expectorant properties help clear mucus, aiding in respiratory health.

Cardiovascular System

Heart: Cardamom can lower blood pressure and improve heart health.

Immune System

Overall Immunity: The spice possesses antimicrobial and antioxidant properties, boosting immune defense.

Skin and Integumentary System

Skin: Its antibacterial properties help in treating skin infections and improving complexion.

Nervous System

Brain: Cardamom's invigorating scent has a refreshing effect that can alleviate stress and enhance mental clarity.

How to Grow Cardamom

- **Selecting the Right Variety:** Cardamom comes in green and black varieties, with green being the most commonly cultivated for its culinary and medicinal value. It's preferable to start with seedlings rather than seeds, as they are easier to manage and grow. Purchase quality seedlings from reputable nurseries or online stores specializing in spice plants.
- **Best Time to Plant Outdoors:** Plant cardamom in the late spring to early summer when the risk of frost has passed, and the soil is warm.
- **Spacing Outdoor Plants:** Space plants about 2 to 3 feet apart to allow for adequate air circulation and growth.
- **Container Use and Soil:** Use large containers with well-draining soil rich in organic matter. A mix of potting soil, compost, and perlite is ideal for container growth.
- **Sunlight and Location:** Cardamom prefers partial shade or filtered sunlight, requiring about 4 to 6 hours of light daily. In hotter climates, provide some afternoon shade to prevent scorching.
- **Watering:** Keep the soil consistently moist but not waterlogged. Water when the top inch of soil feels dry to the touch.
- **Feeding:** Fertilize with a balanced organic fertilizer every 4-6 weeks during the growing season.
- **Pruning and Maintenance:** Regularly snip off dead flowers to encourage more growth and remove any yellowing leaves to maintain plant health.
- **Pest and Disease Management:** Watch for signs of pests like aphids and spider mites, and diseases such as root rot. Use organic pesticides and ensure good drainage to prevent these problems.

- **Overwintering:** In colder climates, overwinter cardamom plants indoors or in a greenhouse to protect them from frost.
- **Propagation:** Propagate cardamom from division of large clumps or by seed in controlled conditions like a greenhouse.
- **Harvesting:** Harvest cardamom pods when they are plump and green before they split open. Dry the pods to preserve flavor.
- **Climate Considerations:** Cardamom thrives in warm, humid, and tropical climates but can be grown in temperate zones with protective measures against cold weather.

How to Use Cardamom

Herbal Teas or Infusions: Soak cardamom seeds or pods in hot water to make a flavorful tea that aids digestion and relieves flatulence.

Tinctures: Cardamom can be used to prepare tinctures, offering digestive and anti-inflammatory benefits.

Salves-Topical Applications: Ground cardamom mixed with a base cream can be applied to the skin to improve complexion and soothe irritations.

Compresses: A compress made with cardamom-infused water can reduce skin inflammation and headaches when applied topically.

Aromatherapy & Essential Oils: Cardamom essential oil, used in aromatherapy, can help with respiratory issues, mental clarity, and emotional well-being.

Herbal Baths: Adding cardamom to bath water can create a soothing herbal bath that relieves stress and skin irritations.

Steam Inhalation: Inhaling steam infused with cardamom can clear nasal passages and improve respiratory health.

Decoctions: A cardamom decoction can be prepared for treating colds, coughs, and to boost the immune system.

Syrups: Cardamom syrup can soothe sore throats and improve cough symptoms.

Gargles & Mouthwashes: Cardamom acts as a natural breath freshener and can be used in gargles or mouthwash to combat oral bacteria.

Powders: Powder from cardamom is used in cooking and as a spice remedy for digestive problems.

Juices: Can also be added to juices for flavor and its carminative (digestive-helping) properties.

Culinary Uses: Cardamom is widely used in cooking and baking, enhancing dishes with its distinctive flavor while providing digestive benefits.

Ease to Grow: 5-7, Medium Maintenance

Growing cardamom requires some attention, particularly in terms of climate and watering needs. It thrives in humid, tropical environments but can be grown in greenhouses or indoors in temperate areas with the right care. Regular watering and protection from extreme temperatures are crucial for healthy growth.

Catnip

Scientifically known as Nepeta Cataria, is a perennial herb famous for its sedative effects on cats but also has numerous benefits for humans.

It's part of the mint family, characterized by its aromatic leaves and tendency to thrive in sunny, dry environments.

Nervous System

Brain: Catnip can alleviate stress and anxiety, promoting relaxation and a sense of calm.

Nerves: It may help reduce nervousness and improve sleep quality due to its mild sedative properties.

Digestive System

Stomach: Catnip aids in digestion, can relieve stomach cramps, and reduce gas and bloating.

Intestines: It helps soothe intestinal inflammation and regulate smooth muscle function in the digestive tract.

Respiratory System

Lungs: Catnip acts as an expectorant, helping clear mucus and ease coughing.

Airways: Can reduce the severity of asthma symptoms and alleviate respiratory congestion.

How to Grow Catnip

- **Selecting the Right Variety:** Catnip, or Nepeta Cataria, comes in several varieties. While the common catnip is most widely used for its effects on cats and medicinal properties, other varieties like lemon catnip offer unique scents and flavors. It's generally best to start with plants or cuttings, as seeds can be slow to germinate. Nurseries or online stores are good places to find quality plants.

- **Best Time to Plant Outdoors:** Spring is the ideal time to plant catnip outdoors, after the last frost has passed. This gives the plant ample time to establish itself before winter.
- **Spacing Outdoor Plants:** Space catnip plants about 18 to 24 inches apart to allow for adequate air circulation and growth.
- **Container Use and Soil:** Catnip grows well in containers, making it a good choice for balconies or indoor gardens. Use well-draining soil and ensure pots have drainage holes to prevent waterlogging.
- **Sunlight and Location:** Catnip thrives in full sun, requiring at least six hours of direct sunlight daily. However, it can tolerate partial shade, especially in hotter climates.
- **Watering:** Water catnip regularly, but let the soil dry out between watering to prevent over-watering and root rot.
- **Feeding:** Catnip doesn't require much fertilizer. A light feeding in spring with a general-purpose fertilizer is sufficient.
- **Pruning and Maintenance:** Regularly snip off dead flowers (deadheading) to encourage more blooms and prevent the plant from becoming too stemmy.
- **Pest and Disease Management:** Catnip is relatively pest-free, but keep an eye out for common garden pests and treat them with appropriate organic methods.
- **Overwintering:** In colder zones, mulch around the base to protect roots from freezing. Potted plants should be moved indoors or to a sheltered area.
- **Propagation:** Catnip can be easily propagated from cuttings or by dividing mature plants in early spring or fall.
- **Harvesting:** Harvest leaves and flowers as needed, preferably in the morning after the dew has dried for the best concentration of oils. Leaves can be used fresh, dried, or frozen.

- **Climate Considerations:** Catnip grows best in temperate climates characterized by moderate temperatures, well-draining soil, and ample sunlight. It thrives in areas with mild winters and warm summers, making it well-suited for regions with a temperate or warm and dry climate.

How to Use Catnip

Herbal Teas or Infusions: Soak dried catnip leaves in boiling water for a calming, sleep-inducing tea.

Tinctures: Steep catnip in alcohol to extract active compounds for use in small, concentrated doses.

Salves-Topical Applications: Infuse catnip in oils or creams for soothing skin irritations or insect bites.

Compresses: Apply a cloth soaked in catnip tea to areas of the body for relief of headaches or sore muscles.

Aromatherapy & Essential Oils: Use catnip essential oil in a diffuser for stress relief or apply diluted oil topically for its calming effects.

Herbal Baths: Add catnip leaves to bathwater for a relaxing soak, beneficial for skin health and relaxation.

Steam Inhalation: Inhale steam from boiling water infused with catnip leaves to alleviate respiratory congestion.

Decoctions: Boil catnip roots or leaves to create a concentrated liquid for digestive issues.

Syrups: Combine catnip decoction with honey to make a soothing syrup for coughs and colds.

Gargles & Mouthwashes: Use a cooled catnip infusion to soothe sore throats or mouth ulcers.

Powders: Dry and grind catnip leaves to create a powder that can be used in capsules or as a seasoning.

Juices: Crush fresh catnip leaves to extract juice beneficial for skin application.

Culinary Uses: Use catnip leaves sparingly in cooking for a minty flavor in salads and sauces.

Ease to Grow: 2-4, Low Maintenance

Catnip is an easy-to-grow plant, thriving in well-draining soil with full sun to partial shade. It's robust, drought-resistant, and grows prolifically, often requiring minimal care beyond basic watering and occasional trimming. Its hardiness and ability to self-seed make it a low-maintenance choice for gardeners.

Cat's Claw

Known scientifically as Uncaria Tomentosa, is a vine commonly found in the rainforests of South America, traditionally used for its health-promoting properties. The plant is named for its claw-shaped thorns and is recognized for its immune-boosting, anti-inflammatory, and antioxidant effects. Research has shown that Cat's Claw can positively affect various physiological systems due to its unique alkaloids, phytochemicals, and compounds.

Immune System

White Blood Cells: Cat's Claw enhances the immune response by increasing the production of white blood cells, particularly lymphocytes, which helps the body fight off infections and diseases more effectively.

Thymus: It stimulates the activity of the thymus gland, enhancing the body's ability to generate a more robust immune response.

Digestive System

Intestinal Tract: Cat's Claw has been shown to reduce inflammation in the gastrointestinal tract, aiding in the relief of conditions like gastritis, ulcers, and intestinal infections.

Stomach: Promotes healing of gastric ulcers and reduces stomach inflammation by inhibiting the production of certain acids and enzymes that contribute to ulcer formation.

Cardiovascular System

Blood Vessels: Cat's Claw can help lower blood pressure by acting as a vasodilator, relaxing the walls of blood vessels, thus improving circulation and heart health.

How to Grow Cat's Claw

- **Selecting the Right Variety:** Cat's Claw, Uncaria Tomentosa, is the most common medicinal variety. It's typically grown from seeds or cuttings. You can purchase these from specialty online retailers or nurseries focusing on medicinal plants. Ensuring you get the right species is crucial for its medicinal properties.
- **Best Time to Plant Outdoors:** The ideal time to plant Cat's Claw outdoors is in the spring, after the threat of frost has passed, to give the plant a full growing season to establish.

- **Spacing Outdoor Plants:** Plant Cat's Claw at least 15-20 feet apart as it grows into a large vine and needs space to spread.
- **Container Use and Soil:** Use large containers with well-draining soil rich in organic matter. The soil should mimic its natural habitat, which is loamy and slightly acidic to neutral.
- **Sunlight and Location:** Prefers partial shade but can tolerate full sun if kept moist. In indoor or greenhouse settings, use full-spectrum grow lights to simulate natural sunlight conditions.
- **Watering:** Keep the soil consistently moist but not waterlogged. Cat's Claw requires a lot of water, especially in dry and hot conditions.
- **Feeding:** Fertilize with a balanced, slow-release fertilizer in the early growing season to support vigorous growth and vine development.
- **Pruning and Maintenance:** Regularly snip off dead flowers to encourage more growth and prevent the vine from becoming too heavy and unmanageable.
- **Pest and Disease Management:** Watch for signs of fungal diseases, such as powdery mildew, and treat with appropriate fungicides. Ensure good air circulation around the plant to reduce the risk of disease.
- **Overwintering:** In colder climates, protect the base of the plant with mulch or bring containers indoors during winter to prevent freezing.
- **Propagation:** Propagate by seeds or cuttings in early spring. Cuttings can be rooted in water or soil to establish new plants.
- **Harvesting:** Harvest the bark and roots of Cat's Claw in the dry season when active compounds are concentrated. Use

clean, sharp tools to cut sections of the vine without harming the main plant.

- **Climate Considerations:** Thrives in warm, humid climates with regular rainfall. It can tolerate short dry periods but prefers consistent moisture throughout the growing season.

How to Use Cat's Claw

Herbal Teas or Infusions: Cat's Claw bark is commonly soaked in hot water to make a tea or infusion. This tea is used to boost the immune system and reduce inflammation.

Tinctures: The bark and roots of Cat's Claw are often used to make tinctures. These concentrated extracts are taken in small doses to support immune health and relieve arthritis symptoms.

Salves-Topical Applications: Cat's Claw can be used in salves or creams for its anti-inflammatory properties, applied topically to relieve joint pain and skin irritations.

Decoctions: A decoction is made by boiling Cat's Claw bark in water for an extended period. This process extracts a higher concentration of the plant's medicinal compounds, used to enhance immune function and treat various health conditions.

Ease to Grow: 4-6, Medium Maintenance

Cat's Claw can be somewhat challenging to grow outside its native environment, requiring attention to mimic the tropical conditions it thrives in, including warmth, humidity, and indirect sunlight.

Chamomile

Known for its daisy-like flowers and apple-like aroma, Chamomile has been a treasured herbal remedy for centuries. Its gentle calming effects make it a popular choice in herbal teas. Chamomile is especially renowned for its benefits to the digestive and nervous systems, but it also offers advantages for the skin.

Digestive System

Stomach: Chamomile tea soothes stomach aches and eases digestion, reducing bloating and discomfort.

Intestines: It can relieve intestinal spasms and acts as a mild laxative, improving bowel movements.

Nervous System

Brain: Chamomile is known to reduce stress and anxiety, promoting relaxation and better sleep.

Nerves: It helps to soothe nervous tension and may alleviate headaches related to stress.

Skin and Integumentary System

Skin: Chamomile's anti-inflammatory properties make it beneficial for treating skin irritations, eczema, and wounds. It can accelerate healing and reduce inflammation.

How to Grow Chamomile

- **Selecting the Right Variety:** Chamomile comes in two common types: German (Matricaria Recutita) and Roman (Chamaemelum Nobile). German chamomile is an annual plant that is commonly used for tea and grows easily from seeds, while Roman chamomile is a perennial ground cover. Seeds are available at garden centers and online seed stores. Starting with seeds is generally preferred, as it is cost-effective and allows for better control over plant health.
- **Best Time to Plant Outdoors:** Plant chamomile seeds in spring after the last frost. The growing season extends through late spring and early summer, offering a window for sowing.
- **Spacing Outdoor Plants:** Space the plants or seeds about 6 to 8 inches apart to allow enough room for growth.
- **Container Use and Soil:** Chamomile thrives in well-drained soil with a neutral pH. When grown in containers, use a potting mix that includes compost to ensure adequate nutrient content and drainage.
- **Sunlight and Location:** This herb prefers full sun but can tolerate partial shade. It needs around 6 hours of sunlight daily. If growing indoors, use grow lights to provide sufficient light.
- **Watering:** Water chamomile regularly but allow the soil to dry out between waterings to prevent over-saturation and root rot.
- **Feeding:** Chamomile does not require frequent fertilization. A light application of organic compost in the growing season can support its growth.
- **Pruning and Maintenance:** Snip off dead flowers to promote more blooms and prevent the plant from seeding all over the garden.

- **Pest and Disease Management:** Chamomile is relatively hardy but watch for aphids and fungal diseases like powdery mildew. Treat with natural pesticides and ensure good air circulation to prevent these issues.
- **Overwintering:** In colder climates, mulch around the plants to protect them from freezing temperatures if you are growing a perennial variety.
- **Propagation:** Easily propagated by seed, chamomile can also be divided in spring or autumn to create new plants.
- **Harvesting:** Harvest chamomile flowers when they are fully open, usually in mid-summer. Use the flowers fresh or dry them for later use in teas, infusions, or other remedies.
- **Climate Considerations:** Chamomile is adaptable but grows best in temperate climates. It can tolerate light frost but thrives in warm, sunny conditions.

How to Use Chamomile

Herbal Teas or Infusions: Soak dried chamomile flowers in hot water for a soothing tea that aids digestion and promotes relaxation.

Tinctures: Chamomile flowers are steeped in alcohol to create a tincture, used to relieve anxiety, inflammation, and digestive issues.

Salves-Topical Applications: Infused in creams or ointments, chamomile treats skin irritations, wounds, and burns due to its anti-inflammatory properties.

Compresses: A cloth soaked in chamomile tea and applied to the skin reduces inflammation and soothes skin conditions.

Aromatherapy & Essential Oils: Chamomile oil, used in diffusers or applied directly, alleviates stress, insomnia, and skin irritations.

Herbal Baths: Adding chamomile to bathwater soothes skin irritations and promotes relaxation.

Steam Inhalation: Inhaling chamomile steam can relieve respiratory conditions and sinus issues.

Decoctions: A concentrated chamomile decoction can be used to soothe gastrointestinal problems.

Syrups: Chamomile syrup soothes coughs and sore throats.

Gargles & Mouthwashes: Chamomile-infused gargles relieve oral inflammation and gum diseases.

Powders: Dried chamomile flowers ground into powder can be used in capsules or as a spice.

Juices: Fresh chamomile juice, though less common, can be consumed for its health benefits.

Culinary Uses: Chamomile flowers can add flavor to teas, desserts, and savory dishes.

Ease to Grow: 2-4, Low Maintenance

Chamomile is easy to grow, thriving in well-drained soil and full sun to partial shade. It requires minimal maintenance, making it suitable for novice gardeners. Regular watering and occasional pruning to remove spent flowers will keep it healthy and productive.

Chaste Tree

Also known as Vitex Agnus-Castus, is a plant renowned for its medicinal properties, particularly in relation to the reproductive and endocrine systems. Its berries, leaves, and flowers have been used for centuries in traditional medicine to treat various ailments. Chaste Tree may also have ancillary effects on other physiological systems, but the most documented and significant benefits are in the below areas.

Reproductive System

Ovaries: Chaste Tree berries help to regulate ovarian functions and alleviate symptoms of premenstrual syndrome (PMS).

Uterus: The plant's extracts are used to treat menstrual cycle irregularities and ease uterine cramps.

Endocrine System

Pituitary Gland: Chaste Tree influences the pituitary gland, helping to normalize hormone levels, especially progesterone and estrogen. This is beneficial for women with hormonal imbalances.

How to Grow Chaste Tree

- **Selecting the Right Variety:** Chaste Tree has several varieties like 'Shoal Creek' and 'Silver Spire'. Choose based on size and bloom color preference. Start with seeds or young plants, available at nurseries or online garden shops. Each variety has its own growth characteristics and climate preferences.
- **Best Time to Plant Outdoors:** Plant in early spring after the last frost. Chaste Tree thrives in warm temperatures and establishes best when given time to acclimate before the heat of summer.
- **Spacing Outdoor Plants:** Space plants 15 to 20 feet apart to accommodate their wide spread at maturity.
- **Container Use and Soil:** Prefers well-draining soil with a neutral to slightly alkaline pH. In containers, use a loamy,

well-draining potting mix and ensure the pot has good drainage holes.

- **Sunlight and Location:** Requires full sun, at least 6 to 8 hours daily. Can tolerate partial shade but blooms best in full sun. For artificial lighting, use full-spectrum grow lights.
- **Watering:** Water deeply but infrequently to establish a strong root system. Mature plants are drought tolerant.
- **Feeding:** Apply a balanced, slow-release fertilizer in early spring to support growth and flowering.
- **Pruning and Maintenance:** Snip off dead flowers to promote new growth and maintain shape. Prune heavily in late winter or early spring to encourage branching.
- **Pest and Disease Management:** Monitor for spider mites and aphids. Treat with neem oil or insecticidal soap as needed. Prevent root rot by ensuring soil is well-draining.
- **Overwintering:** In colder zones, mulch around the base to protect roots from freezing. May die back in winter and regrow in spring.
- **Propagation:** Propagate by seed in fall or by semi-hardwood cuttings in summer.
- **Harvesting:** Harvest leaves and flowers in the morning after dew has dried. Use fresh or dry for later use. Roots and seeds can also be collected.
- **Climate Considerations:** The Chaste Tree grows best in climates with warm to hot summers, mild winters, and consistent rainfall throughout the year. It prefers regions where temperatures do not drop too low in winter and where there is adequate moisture to support its growth.

How to Use Chaste Tree

Herbal Teas or Infusions: Soak the dried leaves or flowers in hot water to make a soothing tea, which can help with hormonal balance and menstrual discomfort.

Tinctures: Extracted from the berries, leaves, or flowers, chaste tree tinctures are used for hormonal regulation and easing PMS symptoms.

Salves-Topical Applications: The leaves or berries can be infused into oils to make creams or ointments, applied topically to alleviate skin irritations and inflammation.

Decoctions: Boil the roots or leaves to create a strong decoction, often used for digestive and liver health.

Powders: Dried and ground parts of the plant, like berries or leaves, can be made into powders for use in capsules or as dietary supplements.

Ease to Grow: 3-5, Low to Medium Maintenance

Growing a Chaste tree is relatively easy, requiring minimal care once established. It adapts well to various soil types and prefers full sun. Regular pruning helps maintain its shape and promotes healthy growth. It's drought-resistant, making it suitable for low-maintenance gardens

Chicory

A plant with bright blue flowers that is more than just ornamental. Known for its bitter roots, it's used in traditional medicine and as a coffee substitute. Its roots, leaves, and flowers all have medicinal properties.

Digestive System

Stomach: Chicory root acts as an appetite stimulant and aids in digestion by increasing bile production.
Liver: Supports liver health by promoting bile secretion, enhancing liver detoxification processes.

Cardiovascular System

Blood vessels: Chicory contains inulin, which can help reduce bad cholesterol levels, protecting against vascular diseases.

Immune System

Overall immunity: Chicory's high antioxidant content strengthens the immune system by combating free radicals.

Endocrine System

Pancreas: Chicory root may help in managing blood sugar levels by modulating insulin resistance.

How to Grow Chicory

- **Selecting the Right Variety:** Chicory comes in several varieties, including the common chicory and radicchio. Seeds are commonly used for planting, available at garden centers and online stores. Choose a variety based on your climate and soil type, as some are better suited for colder or warmer conditions.

- **Best Time to Plant Outdoors:** Plant chicory seeds in early spring or late summer. In cooler climates, early Spring planting gives the plant time to establish before winter.
- **Spacing Outdoor Plants:** Space seeds or starts about 6 to 8 inches apart in rows, with rows spaced 12 to 18 inches apart to allow for growth and air circulation.
- **Container Use and Soil:** Chicory can grow in containers if space is limited. Use well-draining soil rich in organic matter, with a pH of 6.5 to 7.0 for optimal growth.
- **Sunlight and Location:** Requires full sun, with at least 6 hours of direct sunlight daily. If growing indoors, use grow lights to supplement natural light.
- **Watering:** Water regularly, keeping the soil consistently moist but not waterlogged. Reduce watering as the plant matures and during cooler weather.
- **Feeding:** Apply a balanced, slow-release fertilizer at planting and mid-season to support growth and root development.
- **Pruning and Maintenance:** Snip off dead flowers to encourage more growth and prevent the plant from becoming leggy (or stemmy).
- **Pest and Disease Management:** Watch for common pests like aphids and slugs. Use natural remedies, such as neem oil, to treat infestations. Keep the area weed-free to reduce disease risk.
- **Overwintering:** In colder climates, mulch around the base to protect roots from freezing temperatures.
- **Propagation:** Propagate by seed in spring or by dividing root clumps in the autumn.
- **Harvesting:** Roots can be harvested in the second year after planting when they are thick and fleshy, typically in late fall. Leaves and flowers can be picked throughout the growing season as needed.

- **Climate Considerations:** Thrives in temperate climates with cool summers and mild winters, avoiding extreme heat or cold.

How to Use Chicory

Herbal Teas or Infusions: Soak chicory root in hot water to make a coffee-like beverage, known for its digestive benefits and prebiotic properties.

Tinctures: The roots are used to make tinctures that support liver function and aid digestion.

Salves-Topical Applications: Ground chicory root, mixed with a base cream or oil, can be applied to the skin to reduce inflammation.

Compresses: A chicory compress can be made by soaking a cloth in a strong chicory infusion and applied to skin areas to soothe irritation.

Herbal Baths: Adding chicory leaves or flowers to a bath can help with skin problems and promote relaxation.

Steam Inhalation: Inhaling steam from a decoction of chicory can help clear nasal passages and relieve respiratory discomfort.

Decoctions: A chicory root decoction can be used to aid digestion and stimulate the liver.

Syrups: Chicory root syrup, often combined with other herbs, can be used to soothe coughs and sore throats.

Gargles & Mouthwashes: A chicory infusion can be used as a gargle or mouthwash to help with oral health issues.

Powders: Dried chicory root can be ground into a powder and used as a dietary supplement.

Juices: Fresh chicory leaves can be juiced and consumed for their health benefits.

Culinary Uses: Chicory leaves can be used in salads, and the roots can be roasted and ground as a coffee substitute.

Ease to Grow: 3-5, Low to Medium Maintenance

Chicory is relatively easy to grow, adapting well to various soil types and environmental conditions. It requires minimal maintenance, making it suitable for beginner gardeners. The plant thrives in full sun and needs regular watering, but is generally robust and resilient against pests and diseases.

Chives

A member of the onion family, are not only valued for their distinctive flavor but also for their health benefits. These perennial herbs are rich in vitamins and minerals, and have long been used traditionally to aid digestion and boost immunity. Their mild onion taste enhances culinary dishes without overpowering them.

Digestive System

Stomach: Chives stimulate digestion, promoting efficient breakdown and absorption of food, leading to better gastrointestinal health.
Intestines: Help maintain a healthy gut flora, reducing bloating and supporting regular bowel movements.

Immune System

Lymphatic tissue: Chives enhance immune function by providing essential nutrients that support the lymphatic system's role in detoxification and infection defense.

Cardiovascular System

Blood vessels: The sulfur compounds in chives may help lower blood pressure and cholesterol levels, contributing to cardiovascular health.

Reproductive System

Ovaries and Testes: Chives are thought to have a mild stimulating effect on the reproductive organs, supporting their function.

How to Grow Chives

- **Selecting the Right Variety:** Chives come in several varieties, with common chives and garlic chives being the most popular. Common chives offer a mild onion flavor, while garlic chives provide a garlicky taste. It's preferable to start with seeds or starts, available at nurseries or online garden centers.
- **Best Time to Plant Outdoors:** Early spring is the best time to plant chives outdoors, after the last frost, when the soil is workable.
- **Spacing Outdoor Plants:** Plant chives 8 to 12 inches apart to allow enough room for growth and air circulation.
- **Container Use and Soil:** Chives thrive in well-draining soil with a pH of 6 to 7. They are excellent for container gardening, needing pots with good drainage.
- **Sunlight and Location:** Chives require full sun, at least 6 hours of direct sunlight per day. If using artificial lighting, fluorescent or LED grow lights are suitable.
- **Watering:** Keep the soil consistently moist but not waterlogged. Water chives when the top inch of soil feels dry.

- **Feeding:** Apply a balanced liquid fertilizer every 4-6 weeks during the growing season to support their growth.
- **Pruning and Maintenance:** Regularly snip off dead flowers to encourage more leaf production and prevent self-seeding.
- **Pest and Disease Management:** Chives are generally pest-resistant but watch for onion flies and thrips (pesty little bugs). Control pests using organic insecticides or by encouraging beneficial insects.
- **Overwintering:** In colder climates, mulch around the base to protect roots from freezing temperatures.
- **Propagation:** Easily propagated by division in spring or fall, separating clumps every 3-4 years to maintain vigor.
- **Harvesting:** Harvest chive leaves as needed by cutting them at the base. Young leaves have the best flavor. Flowers are also edible and can be used to garnish dishes.
- **Climate Considerations:** Chives grow best in temperate climates with well-defined seasons. They are hardy and can tolerate a wide range of weather conditions but prefer cooler temperatures over extreme heat.

How to Use Chives

Herbal Teas or Infusions: Soak chive leaves in hot water to create a mild, onion-flavored tea, beneficial for digestion and relaxation.
Culinary Uses: Chives are widely used in cooking for their mild onion flavor. They are added to soups, salads, sauces, omelets, and potato dishes, often as a garnish to enhance the flavor.

Ease to Grow: 2-3, Low Maintenance

Growing chives is relatively easy, making them a good choice for novice gardeners. They thrive in a variety of conditions and require minimal care once established. With their hardy nature and low maintenance requirements, chives are a simple and rewarding herb to cultivate in the garden. They adapt well to container gardening and can be easily grown indoors with sufficient light.

Cilantro

Also known as Coriandrum Sativum, is an aromatic herb commonly used in culinary dishes worldwide. Its leaves and seeds (coriander) are used to flavor various recipes. Beyond its culinary uses, cilantro is known for its health benefits. It contains antioxidants, vitamins, and minerals that contribute to overall health.

Digestive System

Stomach: Cilantro can help soothe an upset stomach, reduce nausea, and prevent gas and bloating.

Intestines: Aids in digestion by stimulating digestive enzymes and juices, which enhances the breakdown of food.

Nervous System

Brain: Cilantro contains compounds that can help the brain to enhance the release of calming chemicals, helping to reduce stress and promote relaxation.

Immune System

Lymphatic tissue: Cilantro supports the immune system by offering high levels of antioxidants that combat harmful molecules and lessen cellular damage. It also has antimicrobial properties that help fend off infections and boost overall immunity.

Skin and Integumentary System

Skin: Cilantro benefits the skin by reducing inflammation, which helps soothe irritations and decrease redness. Its antioxidants also protect against UV rays and environmental pollutants, improving skin health.

How to Grow Cilantro

- **Selecting the Right Variety:** Cilantro has varieties like 'Santo' and 'Leisure' that are slow to take off. It's generally started from seeds as transplants can struggle to adapt. Seeds are available at nurseries or online garden stores.
- **Best Time to Plant Outdoors:** Plant cilantro in the spring or fall to avoid hot temperatures that can cause it to grow too rapidly. In cooler climates, you can grow it throughout the summer.
- **Spacing Outdoor Plants:** Space cilantro plants 6 to 8 inches apart to allow enough room for growth.
- **Container Use and Soil:** Cilantro grows well in containers; use well-draining potting mix to prevent waterlogged soil.
- **Sunlight and Location:** Cilantro prefers 6 to 8 hours of direct sunlight but can tolerate partial shade, especially in hot conditions. If using artificial light, T5 fluorescent or full-spectrum LED grow lights are suitable.

- **Watering:** Keep the soil moist but not waterlogged. Cilantro requires consistent watering, especially in hot, dry weather.
- **Feeding:** Apply a balanced liquid fertilizer every 4 to 6 weeks, but avoid over-fertilizing, which can affect the taste.
- **Pruning and Maintenance:** Snip off dead flowers to encourage more leaf growth and prevent the plant from going to seed too early.
- **Pest and Disease Management:** Watch for common pests like aphids and treat with organic insecticidal soap. Root rot can occur in waterlogged soil, so ensure good drainage.
- **Overwintering:** In colder climates, protect cilantro with mulch or a cold frame (transparent protective covering) during winter.
- **Propagation:** Cilantro can self-seed. Allow some plants to complete their life cycle and produce seeds for the next planting.
- **Harvesting:** Harvest leaves once the plant is 6 inches tall by cutting them at the base. Leaves are most flavorful before the plant flowers.
- **Climate Considerations:** Thrives in cooler climates but can be grown in warm areas if provided with shade and adequate water. Avoid extreme heat as it causes the plant to flower too early.

How to Use Cilantro

Herbal Teas or Infusions: Soak cilantro leaves in hot water to make a detoxifying herbal tea, which aids in digestion and can help settle the stomach.

Tinctures: Cilantro tincture can be made by soaking the leaves in alcohol, used for its digestive and anti-inflammatory benefits.

Salves-Topical Applications: Crushed cilantro leaves are often mixed with a carrier oil to create a salve that can soothe skin irritations and inflammation.

Compresses: A compress made from cilantro-infused water can be applied to the skin to alleviate discomfort from minor irritations and burns.

Herbal Baths: Adding cilantro leaves to bathwater can create a refreshing herbal bath that helps to soothe skin conditions and promote relaxation.

Steam Inhalation: Inhaling steam infused with cilantro can relieve respiratory congestion and headaches.

Decoctions: A decoction made from cilantro seeds aids in relieving digestive issues and is sometimes used as a diuretic.

Syrups: Cilantro syrup can easily be made for use in soothing coughs and sore throats.

Gargles & Mouthwashes: A cilantro-based gargle can help freshen breath and has antimicrobial properties that may benefit oral health.

Powders: Dried and powdered cilantro leaves or seeds can be used in cooking and as a spice that promotes digestive health.

Juices: Juice made from cilantro leaves is often consumed for its detoxifying properties.

Culinary Uses: Widely used in cooking for its aromatic flavor, cilantro leaves and seeds add freshness and zest to various dishes and support digestion.

Ease to Grow: 2-3, Low Maintenance

Cilantro is relatively easy to grow, thriving in cool to moderate climates. It requires regular watering and partial shade in hotter regions. With its quick growth cycle, cilantro can be harvested just a few weeks after planting. Being low maintenance, it's suitable for beginners and does not demand extensive care.

Cinnamon

Derived from the inner bark of trees in the genus Cinnamomum, is a spice that has been valued for its medicinal properties for thousands of years. It contains 'cinnamaldehyde", which is responsible for its distinct flavor and health benefits. Cinnamon is known for its potent antioxidant, anti-inflammatory, and antimicrobial effects. It's commonly used in traditional medicine and has been studied for its impact on various physiological systems.

Digestive System

Stomach: Cinnamon stimulates digestive enzymes, which aids in breaking down food more efficiently and relieves indigestion.
Intestines: Has been shown to improve intestinal health by reducing inflammation and combating bacterial infections.

Cardiovascular System

Blood vessels: Cinnamon can reduce blood pressure and improve circulation by relaxing the blood vessel walls.
Heart: Also known to reduce cholesterol levels, thus lowering the risk of heart disease.

Immune System

Immune cells: The antimicrobial and anti-inflammatory properties of cinnamon strengthen the immune response against pathogens.

Endocrine System

Pancreas: Cinnamon has been noted to enhance insulin sensitivity and regulate blood sugar levels, benefiting those with type 2 diabetes.

How to Grow Cinnamon

- **Selecting the Right Variety:** Cinnamon is derived from the bark of the Cinnamomum Verum tree, also known as "true cinnamon" or Ceylon cinnamon. Another common type is Cassia cinnamon from Cinnamomum cassia. It's preferable to start with young plants or cuttings rather than seeds, as growing from seeds can be challenging and time-consuming. These plants are usually sourced from specialized nurseries or online stores that offer tropical plants.

- **Best Time to Plant Outdoors:** The best time to plant cinnamon is during the spring or early summer in tropical or subtropical climates to ensure the plant has enough time to establish before cooler temperatures.

- **Spacing Outdoor Plants:** Space plants at least 10 feet apart to allow room for growth, as cinnamon trees can grow quite large.

- **Container Use and Soil:** Cinnamon can be grown in large containers using well-draining soil rich in organic matter. Ensure your pot has adequate drainage holes.

- **Sunlight and Location:** Requires partial to full sunlight, around 4-6 hours of direct sunlight daily. If using artificial lighting, full-spectrum grow lights are recommended.

- **Watering:** Keep the soil consistently moist but not waterlogged. Reduce watering during the cooler months to prevent root rot.
- **Feeding:** Apply a balanced, slow-release fertilizer every few months to support growth.
- **Pruning and Maintenance:** Prune to shape the plant and encourage bushier growth. Snip off dead flowers to prevent the plant from flowering too early.
- **Pest and Disease Management:** Watch for common pests like aphids and spider mites. Treat diseases like root rot by ensuring good drainage and not overwatering.
- **Overwintering:** In cooler climates, protect the plant from frost by bringing containers indoors or using frost covers outdoors.
- **Propagation:** Best propagated through cuttings or layering to ensure the characteristics of the parent plant are maintained.
- **Harvesting:** Bark can be harvested from trees that are at least 2-3 years old. The best time to harvest is during the dry season when the bark peels off easily.
- **Climate Considerations:** Thrives in warm, humid environments with regular rainfall. Areas with a tropical climate are ideal, avoiding extreme temperature fluctuations.

How to Use Cinnamon

Herbal Teas or Infusions: Soak cinnamon bark in hot water to create a soothing, aromatic tea that can aid digestion and provide antioxidants.

Tinctures: Cinnamon bark is soaked in alcohol to extract its concentrated flavors and medicinal properties, used for digestive health.

Salves-Topical Applications: Ground cinnamon or oil is mixed into creams or ointments for antimicrobial and anti-inflammatory skin treatments.

Compresses: A cloth soaked in cinnamon-infused water is applied to the skin to relieve inflammation and pain.

Aromatherapy & Essential Oils: Cinnamon essential oil is used in diffusers for its warm, stimulating scent or applied topically when diluted for pain relief.

Herbal Baths: Adding cinnamon to bathwater can provide a relaxing experience and skin benefits due to its antimicrobial properties.

Steam Inhalation: Inhaling steam infused with cinnamon oil can relieve respiratory congestion and soothe the airways.

Decoctions: Boiling cinnamon bark creates a strong decoction used for medicinal purposes, especially for gastrointestinal issues.

Syrups: Cinnamon is added to syrups for flavor and its soothing effects on the throat and digestive system.

Gargles & Mouthwashes: Cinnamon's antibacterial properties make it effective in mouthwashes and gargles for oral health.

Powders: Cinnamon powder is used in food preparations and as a spice for its health benefits and flavor.

Juices: Cinnamon is sometimes added to juices to enhance flavor and provide metabolic benefits.

Culinary Uses: Widely used in cooking and baking for its distinct flavor and aroma, cinnamon also offers antioxidant benefits.

Ease to Grow: 6-8, Medium Maintenance

Growing cinnamon requires a warm, humid climate and consistent care. It needs well-draining soil, regular watering, and protection from cold temperatures. Harvesting the bark involves labor-intensive processes, making it medium maintenance. The plant is best suited for tropical climates or controlled environments like greenhouses.

Clove

A perennial evergreen plant, is renowned for its aromatic flower buds used in both culinary and medicinal contexts. Originating from the Maluku Islands in Indonesia, clove has been a global commodity for centuries. It contains eugenol, a compound with potent antiseptic and anesthetic properties, making it popular in traditional medicine.

Digestive System

Stomach: Clove stimulates digestion, increases gastric secretions, and reduces nausea and upset stomach.

Intestines: Its antiseptic properties help in controlling intestinal parasites, infections, and inflammation.

Immune System

Lymph nodes: Clove's eugenol content strengthens immune defenses and fights infections.

Respiratory System

Lungs: Clove acts as an expectorant, helping to clear mucus and relieve coughing.

Bronchi: Its anti-inflammatory properties reduce bronchial inflammation and ease breathing.

Nervous System

Brain: Clove oil is thought to have a stimulating effect, enhancing concentration and reducing mental fatigue.

Skin and Integumentary System

Skin: Clove oil's antiseptic properties make it useful for treating skin infections and wounds.

How to Grow Clove

- **Selecting the Right Variety:** Clove trees (Syzygium Aromaticum) are the source of clove buds. There is primarily one main variety cultivated, so focus on sourcing healthy, robust seedlings from reputable nurseries or online suppliers. Clove trees are not typically grown from seeds by casual gardeners due to their long maturation period.
- **Best Time to Plant Outdoors:** Plant clove trees during the rainy season in tropical climates, which provides the moisture needed for establishment. In temperate regions, plant in late spring to early summer to avoid frost damage.
- **Spacing Outdoor Plants:** Space clove trees 20 to 30 feet apart to accommodate their canopy spread and root growth.
- **Container Use and Soil:** While typically grown in the ground, young clove trees can start in large containers with well-draining, fertile soil, rich in organic matter.
- **Sunlight and Location:** Requires full sun to partial shade, with a minimum of 6 hours of sunlight daily. In areas outside their native tropical habitat, use greenhouse facilities to provide controlled conditions.

- **Watering:** Water regularly to keep the soil consistently moist but not waterlogged. Clove trees are sensitive to drought, especially in the growing stage.
- **Feeding:** Apply balanced, slow-release fertilizer every few months during the growing season to support healthy growth.
- **Pruning and Maintenance:** Prune to shape the tree and remove any dead or diseased branches. Snip off dead flowers to promote healthier growth.
- **Pest and Disease Management:** Watch for signs of fungal diseases and pest infestations, such as leaf spot and scale insects. Use organic pesticides and fungicides as necessary.
- **Overwintering:** In cooler climates, protect young trees from frost. Mature clove trees can withstand short cold periods, but prolonged frost is detrimental.
- **Propagation:** Propagated mainly through seeds or cuttings. However, due to long maturation, it's more efficient to purchase seedlings for cultivation.
- **Harvesting:** Harvest cloves when the flower buds are pink and plump, just before they flower, to get the highest concentration of oils. Dry the buds in the sun until they turn brown.
- **Climate Considerations:** Thrives in tropical climates with high humidity and rainfall. Struggles in cold, dry conditions; not suitable for temperate zones without a controlled environment.

How to Use Clove

Herbal Teas or Infusions: Soak clove buds in hot water to create a spicy, aromatic tea that aids digestion and relieves nausea.

Tinctures: Steep clove buds in alcohol to extract their oils, creating a potent tincture for medicinal use, particularly for dental pain relief.

Salves-Topical Applications: Ground cloves are mixed with carrier oils or creams to make ointments that relieve topical pain and reduce inflammation.

Compresses: A cloth soaked in a decoction of clove can be applied to areas of pain or inflammation for relief.

Aromatherapy & Essential Oils: Clove essential oil is used in diffusers for its strong, warming scent, which can reduce respiratory ailments and improve mood.

Herbal Baths: Adding ground clove or its essential oil to bath water can provide a soothing and antimicrobial bathing experience.

Steam Inhalation: Inhaling steam infused with clove essential oil can clear nasal passages and relieve respiratory conditions.

Decoctions: Boiling cloves in water makes a strong decoction that can soothe gastrointestinal issues and act as an expectorant.

Syrups: Clove syrup can be made by reducing a clove decoction with sugar, offering a flavorful remedy for coughs and sore throats.

Gargles & Mouthwashes: A clove infusion can be used as a gargle or mouthwash to alleviate toothache, gum pain, and bad breath.

Powders: Dried and powdered clove is used in culinary preparations and as a spice in various dishes for flavor and health benefits.

Culinary Uses: Cloves are commonly used in cooking for their intense flavor, especially in spice blends, meats, and baked goods.

Ease to Grow: 7-9, High Maintenance

Growing clove trees requires a specific tropical environment, consistent care, and patience due to their slow growth and long maturation period. They thrive in warm, humid climates with well-drained soil. Due to these conditions, cultivating cloves can be quite challenging outside tropical regions.

Cumin

Also known as Cuminum Cyminum, is an annual herbaceous plant belonging to the Apiaceae family. Widely recognized for its culinary uses, particularly in spice blends and seasonings due to its distinctively warm, earthy flavor and aroma. Originating from the eastern Mediterranean to South Asia, cumin has been utilized for thousands of years, not only in cooking but also in traditional medicine. Its seeds, both in whole and ground form, are used to flavor various dishes, and contain several beneficial nutrients, including iron, manganese, and other vitamins and minerals.

Digestive System

Stomach: Cumin stimulates digestive enzymes, improving the breakdown of food and nutrient absorption.
Intestines: It promotes healthy gut flora and aids in relieving digestive issues like bloating and gas.

Nervous System

Brain: Cumin contains compounds that might help in improving cognitive performance and memory enhancement.

Immune System

General immune response: The seeds have antioxidants which help in boosting the immune system's effectiveness against infections.

How to Grow Cumin

- **Selecting the Right Variety:** Cumin is typically grown from seeds, and the common variety used is Cuminum Cyminum. You can buy seeds from online retailers or local garden stores. It's best to choose high-quality, organic seeds for optimal growth and flavor.
- **Best Time to Plant Outdoors:** Plant cumin seeds in the spring, after the last frost, when the soil has warmed up.
- **Spacing Outdoor Plants:** Space plants or seeds about 4 to 8 inches apart to ensure adequate airflow and light penetration.
- **Container Use and Soil:** Cumin can be grown in containers using well-draining soil. Ensure the pot has adequate drainage holes to prevent waterlogging.
- **Sunlight and Location:** Cumin thrives in full sunlight, needing at least 6 to 8 hours of direct sun daily. If growing indoors, use grow lights to supplement sunlight.
- **Watering:** Water the plants regularly but allow the soil to dry out between watering to prevent root rot.
- **Feeding:** Apply a balanced, slow-release fertilizer at the beginning of the growing season to support growth.
- **Pruning and Maintenance:** Remove any wilted or dead parts of the plant to encourage healthy growth and air circulation. Snip off dead flowers to prevent the plant from flowering too early.

- **Pest and Disease Management:** Watch for common pests like aphids and spider mites. Treat infestations promptly with appropriate organic pesticides or natural remedies.
- **Overwintering:** Cumin is generally grown as an annual, so overwintering is not applicable.
- **Propagation:** Propagate cumin through seeds. Save some from your harvest to plant the next season.
- **Harvesting:** Harvest cumin seeds when they turn brown and are aromatic, usually a few months after planting. Dry them well before storage.
- **Climate Considerations:** Cumin prefers a warm climate with long, hot summers. It doesn't grow well in cold or very humid conditions. Avoid areas with heavy rainfall or high humidity.

How to Use Cumin

Herbal Teas or Infusions: Soak cumin seeds in hot water to create a digestive aid tea, releasing their spicy, earthy flavor and beneficial oils.

Tinctures: Cumin seeds are infused in alcohol to extract their active compounds, used for their digestive properties.

Salves-Topical Applications: Ground cumin, mixed with a base like beeswax or shea butter, can be applied to the skin to soothe irritations or inflammations.

Decoctions: Boil cumin seeds to concentrate their essence in liquid form, used for treating digestive issues.

Culinary Uses: Cumin is extensively used in cooking for its distinct flavor. It's a staple in spice blends and is used to season a variety of dishes.

Ease to Grow: 3-5, Low to Medium Maintenance

Cumin is relatively easy to grow in suitable climates, requiring full sun and well-drained soil. It needs regular watering but should not be over-watered. Harvesting the seeds at the right time ensures the best flavor and medicinal properties.

Damiana

A shrub native to the southern United States, Central America, and South America, is recognized for its aromatic leaves which are used in traditional medicine. It is particularly noted for its aphrodisiac effects and its ability to boost mental and physical stamina. Damiana has been used historically to alleviate symptoms of depression and anxiety, and to improve digestive health. It is believed to stimulate the digestive system, enhance mood and mental clarity, and support the reproductive system.

Nervous System

Brain: Damiana acts as a mild mood enhancer and may help reduce anxiety and stress, promoting mental well-being.

Digestive System

Stomach: Damiana has been used to relieve stomach aches, improve digestion, and treat constipation, aiding overall digestive health.

Reproductive System

Sexual organs: Traditionally used as an aphrodisiac, it is believed to increase sexual desire and performance.

How to Grow Damiana

- **Selecting the Right Variety:** Damiana typically comes in a single species, Turnera Diffusa. It's best started from seeds or cuttings. Seeds and plants can be purchased online or from specialty herb nurseries.
- **Best Time to Plant Outdoors:** Plant in spring after the last frost. Damiana thrives in warm conditions and should be planted when temperatures consistently exceed 60°F.
- **Spacing Outdoor Plants:** Space plants or seeds about 18 to 24 inches apart to allow for growth and airflow, which prevents disease.
- **Container Use and Soil:** Prefers well-draining soil with a neutral to slightly acidic pH. In containers, use a standard potting mix and ensure pots have good drainage.
- **Sunlight and Location:** Requires full sun, with at least 6 hours of direct sunlight daily. In regions with intense heat, partial afternoon shade can prevent scorching.
- **Watering:** Water regularly to keep the soil moist but not waterlogged. Reduce watering in cooler months to prevent root rot.
- **Feeding:** Feed with a balanced liquid fertilizer monthly during the growing season to encourage lush growth.
- **Pruning and Maintenance:** Snip off dead flowers to promote new growth. Regularly check for and remove any dead or yellowing leaves.

- **Pest and Disease Management:** Monitor for common pests like spider mites and aphids. Treat infestations promptly with organic pesticides. Avoid overwatering to prevent fungal diseases.
- **Overwintering:** In cooler climates, bring potted plants indoors or provide a mulch layer to protect outdoor plants from freezing temperatures.
- **Propagation:** Easily propagated by seeds or cuttings in the late spring or early summer. Ensure cuttings are planted in well-draining soil and kept moist until established.
- **Harvesting:** Leaves and flowers can be harvested as needed. Harvest in the morning after dew has dried for optimal potency. Entire stems can be cut and dried for later use.
- **Climate Considerations:** Thrives in warm, sunny climates similar to its native environment. Not suitable for cold, damp climates without protective measures and prefers regions with a warm, dry season.

How to Use Damiana

Herbal Teas or Infusions: Damiana leaves are soaked in hot water to create a relaxing tea, often used for its calming effects and to enhance mood.

Tinctures: The leaves are soaked in alcohol to extract the active ingredients, creating a potent tincture used for its therapeutic benefits, including libido enhancement.

Salves-Topical Applications: Damiana can be infused in creams or ointments to apply topically, aiding in skin health and for muscle relaxation.

Compresses: A cloth soaked in a damiana infusion can be applied to the skin to soothe and relax affected areas, providing local relief.

Aromatherapy & Essential Oils: Damiana essential oil is used in diffusers or applied directly to the skin when diluted, offering stress relief and mood enhancement.

Herbal Baths: Adding damiana leaves to bathwater can create a soothing herbal bath, promoting relaxation and skin health.

Steam Inhalation: Inhaling the steam from boiled damiana leaves can help clear respiratory passages and relax the mind.

Decoctions: Boiled damiana leaves create a strong decoction, often used for its expectorant and mood-lifting properties.

Syrups: Damiana can be made into a syrup for ease of consumption, often used to enhance digestive health and mood.

Gargles & Mouthwashes: A damiana infusion can be used as a gargle or mouthwash to support oral health and soothe throat discomfort.

Powders: Dried damiana leaves can be ground into a powder, which is used to make capsules for convenient consumption.

Juices: Fresh damiana leaves can be juiced and consumed for their health benefits, including support for the digestive and nervous systems.

Culinary Uses: Although not commonly used in cooking, damiana can be added to dishes for its unique flavor and potential health benefits.

Ease to Grow: 4-6, Medium Maintenance

Damiana is relatively easy to grow in the right climate conditions, preferring warm and sunny environments. It requires regular watering but is drought-resistant once established. This plant is not very demanding but benefits from occasional feeding and pruning to encourage healthy growth.

Dandelion

Scientifically known as Taraxacum Officinale, is a perennial herb with a long history of medicinal use. It's recognized for its yellow flowers, deeply toothed leaves, and ability to grow in diverse climates. Every part of the plant, from root to flower, is edible and packed with vitamins and minerals. Dandelion is known for its detoxifying properties and support of various physiological systems.

Digestive System

Liver: Dandelion supports liver function, aids detoxification, and promotes bile production.

Stomach: Dandelion's bitter compounds stimulate digestive secretions and bile production, aiding in the breakdown of food, improving digestion, and alleviating issues like indigestion and bloating.

Urinary System

Kidneys: Acts as a diuretic, increasing urine production and promoting the elimination of waste, aiding in kidney function and potentially reducing the risk of urinary tract infections and kidney stones.

Cardiovascular System

Blood vessels: Dandelion contains potassium, which can help manage blood pressure by balancing fluid levels in the body, and may also influence the lipid profile, potentially reducing atherosclerosis risk (buildup of plaque).

Endocrine System

Pancreas: Dandelion's potential effect on blood sugar regulation may be due to its role in enhancing insulin sensitivity and promoting glucose metabolism, supporting pancreatic health.

How to Grow Dandelion

- **Selecting the Right Variety:** Dandelion (Taraxacum Officinale) is generally uniform in its variety, but some cultivars may offer larger leaves or roots. It's preferable to start with seeds, which are widely available online or at garden centers. No specific variety recommendation is needed as common dandelion is robust and grows well in most conditions.
- **Best Time to Plant Outdoors:** Early spring is the best time to sow dandelion seeds directly in the garden, as the cool weather helps with germination.
- **Spacing Outdoor Plants:** Space plants or seeds about 6-12 inches apart, as dandelion leaves can spread wide.
- **Container Use and Soil:** Dandelions grow well in containers using any standard potting mix; they are not picky about soil type but prefer a well-draining one.
- **Sunlight and Location:** Dandelions need full sun to partial shade, thriving in both conditions. They require at least 4-6 hours of sunlight per day.

- **Watering:** Water regularly to keep the soil moist but not waterlogged, as dandelions are drought-tolerant once established.
- **Feeding:** Dandelions generally do not require additional fertilization if grown in decent soil.
- **Pruning and Maintenance:** Snip off dead flowers to prevent the plant from spreading excessively. Regular trimming of leaves encourages growth.
- **Pest and Disease Management:** Dandelions are hardy and face few pest or disease issues. Monitor for common garden pests and treat naturally if needed.
- **Overwintering:** Dandelions are perennials that naturally die back in winter and re-sprout in spring. No special overwintering care is needed.
- **Propagation:** Easily propagated by seeds, which will self-sow. You can collect seeds from spent flowers to plant in new areas if desired.
- **Harvesting:** All parts of the dandelion can be harvested - roots, leaves, and flowers. Leaves are best picked in spring when tender, roots in fall, and flowers whenever they are in bloom. Each part has its uses, from salads to teas to topical applications.
- **Climate Considerations:** Dandelions are incredibly adaptable and can grow in a wide range of climates. They are hardy and can tolerate varying temperatures, making them suitable for most growing conditions except for extreme cold or heat.

How to Use Dandelion

Herbal Teas or Infusions: Soak dried dandelion leaves or roots in boiling water to create a detoxifying tea that aids digestion and supports liver function.

Tinctures: Dandelion roots or leaves are macerated in alcohol to extract their beneficial compounds, creating a concentrated tincture that supports digestive health and detoxification.

Salves-Topical Applications: Infused dandelion oil is combined with beeswax to make salves or ointments, applied topically to soothe skin irritations and muscle aches.

Compresses: Dandelion tea or decoction-soaked cloth is applied to the skin to reduce inflammation and soothe skin conditions.

Herbal Baths: Dandelion flowers or leaves are added to bathwater for a relaxing soak that helps alleviate skin problems and muscular pain.

Steam Inhalation: Inhaling steam from a decoction of dandelion leaves or flowers can relieve nasal congestion and respiratory issues.

Decoctions: Boiling dandelion roots or leaves in water makes a strong decoction used for digestive problems and liver detox.

Syrups: Dandelion flowers are simmered with water and sugar to create a syrup that soothes sore throats and coughs.

Gargles & Mouthwashes: A decoction of dandelion can be used as a gargle or mouthwash to treat mouth ulcers and sore throats.

Powders: Dried and ground dandelion leaves or roots are used as a powder supplement to support digestion and liver health.

Juices: Fresh dandelion leaves are juiced and consumed for their detoxifying and nutritional benefits.

Culinary Uses: Dandelion leaves are eaten in salads, roots are roasted and used as a coffee substitute, and flowers are used to make dandelion wine.

Ease to Grow: 1-2, Low Maintenance

Dandelion is extremely easy to grow, thriving in almost any soil and requiring minimal care. It's hardy and self-seeds, often considered a weed because of its ability to spread and grow in diverse environments.

Dong Quai

Also known as Angelica Sinensis, is a revered herb in traditional Chinese medicine, often dubbed the "female ginseng" due to its benefits for women's health. Native to China, it thrives in cool, high-altitude regions and is cultivated for its fragrant, medicinal roots. Dong Quai is recognized for its ability to regulate the menstrual cycle, alleviate menopausal symptoms, and improve blood health.

Reproductive System

Uterus: Dong Quai is known to regulate estrogen levels, improve uterine health, and alleviate menstrual cramps by relaxing uterine muscles.

Hormonal Regulation: Aids in balancing hormone levels, reducing symptoms of menopause like hot flashes and mood swings.

Cardiovascular System

Blood Circulation: Dong Quai acts as a blood tonic, improving circulation and nourishing the blood, which helps in preventing anemia and fatigue.

Blood Vessels: It is believed to dilate blood vessels, lowering blood pressure, and improving overall cardiovascular health.

Nervous System

Brain Function: Dong Quai contains compounds that may support cognitive functions, potentially improving memory and focus.

Stress and Anxiety: It is thought to have a calming effect on the nervous system, helping to alleviate stress and reduce symptoms of anxiety.

Sleep: Potential sedative properties may aid in improving sleep quality and relaxation, helping to combat insomnia.

How to Grow Dong Quai

- **Selecting the Right Variety:** Dong Quai has a few varieties, with Angelica Sinensis being the most commonly used for medicinal purposes. It is preferable to start with seeds, which are available at specialty health stores or online herbal shops. Choose a reputable supplier to ensure quality and viability of the seeds.

- **Best Time to Plant Outdoors:** Plant in early spring, after the last frost, when the soil is workable and warm enough to encourage germination.

- **Spacing Outdoor Plants:** Space plants or seeds about 8 to 12 inches apart to allow enough room for growth and air circulation, which helps prevent disease.

- **Container Use and Soil:** Dong Quai thrives in deep, rich, well-drained soil with a pH of 6.0 to 7.0. If growing in containers, ensure they are deep enough to accommodate the long taproot and use a mix of garden soil and compost.

- **Sunlight and Location:** Prefers partial shade, requiring about 4 to 6 hours of sunlight daily. In areas with strong sun, provide some afternoon shade to protect the plant.

- **Watering:** Keep the soil consistently moist but not waterlogged. Watering is particularly crucial during dry spells to prevent the soil from drying out completely.
- **Feeding:** Fertilize with a balanced, slow-release fertilizer in the spring to support robust growth.
- **Pruning and Maintenance:** Snip off dead flowers to prevent the plant from flowering too early, which can divert energy away from root development.
- **Pest and Disease Management:** Watch for common garden pests and fungal diseases. Maintain healthy soil and adequate spacing to reduce the risk. Treat infestations or infections early with appropriate organic or chemical controls.
- **Overwintering:** In colder regions, mulch heavily around the base to protect the root system from freezing temperatures.
- **Propagation:** Propagate by dividing the root clump in the fall or spring. Seed propagation is also possible but requires patience, as germination can be slow and uneven.
- **Harvesting:** The root is the most valuable part, typically harvested in the fall of the third year when medicinal compounds are at their peak. Carefully dig up the plant, remove the root, clean, and dry it for use.
- **Climate Considerations:** Prefers a temperate climate with cold winters and mild summers. It doesn't thrive in extreme heat or tropical conditions. Ideal climates are those with distinct seasons and moderate summer temperatures.

How to Use Dong Quai

Herbal Teas or Infusions: Dong Quai can be soaked in hot water to make a herbal tea. The roots are sliced or ground before soaking to release their properties, which are believed to support female reproductive health.

Tinctures: The root of Dong Quai is often soaked in alcohol to create a tincture, concentrating its active compounds, which are then used in small doses for therapeutic effects.

Salves-Topical Applications: Ground Dong Quai root can be mixed with creams or ointments to apply on the skin, aiding in the healing of wounds and improving circulation.

Compresses: A cloth soaked in a decoction of Dong Quai can be applied to areas of pain or swelling to reduce symptoms and improve blood flow.

Decoctions: The root is boiled in water to make a strong decoction, often used in traditional medicine to help with menstrual cramps and to balance hormones.

Powders: Dong Quai root is dried and ground into a powder that can be used in capsules or mixed with other herbs in supplements for health benefits.

Culinary Uses: While less common, Dong Quai can be used in small amounts in cooking, especially in soups and herbal dishes, to impart its earthy flavor and health benefits.

Ease to Grow: 3-6, Medium Maintenance

Growing Dong Quai requires some attention to soil, light, and water conditions. It prefers cool, shaded areas and well-drained soil. Although it's not overly demanding, maintaining the right environment for its growth and waiting for the roots to mature can be moderately challenging.

Echinacea

Commonly known as the purple coneflower, is a perennial plant that is well-regarded for its medicinal properties. Originating from North America, it has been used traditionally by Native Americans to treat a variety of ailments. It's distinguished by its tall stems, broad leaves, and large daisy-like flowers with pinkish-purple petals surrounding a spiky, cone-shaped center. Echinacea is most famed for its ability to enhance the immune system. It contains several active compounds such as phenols, alkamides, and polysaccharides, which are thought to increase the body's production of white blood cells and boost immune response.

Immune System

White Blood Cells: Echinacea can stimulate the production of white blood cells, enhancing the body's ability to fight infections more effectively.

Skin and Integumentary System

Skin Healing: Echinacea promotes skin healing, reducing inflammation and aiding in the treatment of wounds, eczema, and other skin conditions..

Respiratory System

Lungs: It may help reduce the symptoms of respiratory conditions like the common cold and bronchitis by supporting lung function and reducing inflammation.

How to Grow Echinacea

- **Selecting the Right Variety:** Echinacea Purpurea, Echinacea Angustifolia, and Echinacea Pallida are beneficial varieties. Starting from seeds or starts is common; seeds may take longer to germinate but are often more cost-effective. Available at nurseries, garden centers, or online.
- **Best Time to Plant Outdoors:** Plant in spring or early fall when the temperature is cooler to allow the plants to establish without the stress of midsummer heat.
- **Spacing Outdoor Plants:** Space plants about 18 to 24 inches apart to ensure adequate air circulation and reduce the risk of disease.
- **Container Use and Soil:** Use well-draining soil with a neutral pH in containers or garden beds. Echinacea thrives in loamy soil but is adaptable to clay or sandy soils if drainage is good.
- **Sunlight and Location:** Prefers full sun, needing at least 6 to 8 hours of direct sunlight daily. Can tolerate partial shade but may flower less.
- **Watering:** Water regularly to establish plants, then reduce frequency. Echinacea is drought-tolerant but benefits from occasional watering during prolonged dry spells.
- **Feeding:** Apply a balanced, slow-release fertilizer in the spring. Excessive feeding can lead to weak growth and fewer flowers.

- **Pruning and Maintenance:** Snip off dead flowers to encourage more blooms and prevent the plant from flowering too early. Cut back stems to the ground in late fall or early spring to promote healthy growth.
- **Pest and Disease Management:** Watch for aphids and powdery mildew. Treat aphids with soapy water or neem oil. Ensure good air circulation and water at the base to prevent powdery mildew.
- **Overwintering:** Mulch around the base in late fall to protect roots in colder climates.
- **Propagation:** Propagate by dividing large clumps in spring or fall or by sowing seeds.
- **Harvesting:** Harvest leaves and flowers in summer when they are in full bloom for medicinal use. Roots can be harvested in the fall of the second or third year.
- **Climate Considerations:** Thrives in temperate climates with cold winters and hot summers. Prefers regions with distinct seasons and can tolerate winter cold well.

How to Use Echinacea

Herbal Teas or Infusions: Echinacea leaves or flowers can be soaked in hot water for 10-15 minutes to make a herbal tea, which is commonly consumed to boost the immune system.

Tinctures: Echinacea can be used to make a tincture by soaking the root or aerial parts in alcohol, which is then used to stimulate the immune system.

Salves-Topical Applications: The plant's extracts are often incorporated into creams or ointments to heal cuts, burns, and skin irritations due to its anti-inflammatory properties.

Compresses: Soaked leaves or flowers applied to the skin can relieve inflammation and treat wounds.

Aromatherapy & Essential Oils: While not commonly used in aromatherapy, echinacea essential oil can be applied topically for its therapeutic properties.

Herbal Baths: Adding echinacea to a bath can help soothe skin issues and promote relaxation.

Steam Inhalation: Inhaling the steam of boiled echinacea can alleviate respiratory conditions.

Decoctions: Boiling the roots to create a strong tea can be used for medicinal purposes, especially for immune support.

Syrups: Echinacea can be made into a syrup, often combined with other herbs, to ease coughs and sore throats.

Gargles & Mouthwashes: A gargle solution made from echinacea extract can help soothe a sore throat and combat oral infections.

Powders: Dried and powdered echinacea can be used in capsules or as a dietary supplement.

Juices: Fresh echinacea juice, extracted from the plant, is sometimes used for its health benefits.

Culinary Uses: Although not commonly used in cooking, the leaves and flowers can be eaten in salads or prepared as a vegetable.

Ease to Grow: 2-4, Low Maintenance

Echinacea is quite easy to grow, requiring minimal care. It thrives in full sun and well-drained soil and is drought-tolerant once established. With its hardy nature, echinacea is a low-maintenance plant ideal for beginner gardeners. It's resilient against pests and diseases, making it a hassle-free addition to any garden.

Elderberry

A plant rich in history and medicinal value, known for its small, dark berries and delicate white flowers. It has been used for centuries in traditional medicine across various cultures to treat a multitude of ailments. Elderberry is especially recognized for its benefits to the immune system, as it is packed with antioxidants and vitamins that boost immunity and combat inflammation. The berries and flowers of the elderberry plant are the most commonly used parts for their health benefits.

Respiratory System
Airways and lungs: Helps alleviate cold and flu symptoms by reducing congestion and soothing the respiratory tract.

Digestive System
Gastrointestinal tract: The fiber in elderberries promotes healthy digestion and can relieve constipation.

Immune System
Immune response: Rich in antioxidants, enhances the body's immune defense against infections.

Skin and Integumentary System

Skin health: Applied topically, elderberry extract can reduce inflammation and treat skin irritations.

How to Grow Elderberry

- **Selecting the Right Variety:** Various types of elderberry include the European elder (Sambucus Nigra) and the American elder (Sambucus Canadensis), with both being popular for their fruit and flowers. Start with seeds or cuttings, available at nurseries or online garden centers.
- **Best Time to Plant Outdoors:** Plant in early spring after the last frost. Elderberry can adapt to different climates but thrives in temperate regions.
- **Spacing Outdoor Plants:** Space plants 6 to 8 feet apart to allow room for growth, as elderberry bushes can grow large.
- **Container Use and Soil:** Prefers well-draining, loamy soil with a pH between 5.5 and 6.5. Can be grown in large containers using a potting mix designed for trees and shrubs.
- **Sunlight and Location:** Requires full sun to partial shade, with at least 6 hours of sunlight per day. If using artificial lighting, full-spectrum LED lights are suitable.
- **Watering:** Keep the soil consistently moist but not waterlogged, especially during dry periods.
- **Feeding:** Apply a balanced fertilizer in early spring and again in mid-summer to support growth and fruit production.
- **Pruning and Maintenance:** Snip off dead flowers to encourage more fruit and prune in late winter to maintain shape and size.
- **Pest and Disease Management:** Watch for signs like wilted leaves or blackened stems, which could indicate disease.

Treat with appropriate fungicides or pesticides and remove affected parts.

- **Overwintering:** In colder climates, mulch around the base to protect roots from freezing temperatures.
- **Propagation:** Propagate by cuttings or by dividing older plants in early spring.
- **Harvesting:** Harvest berries when fully ripe, typically in late summer to early autumn. The flowers can be picked earlier in the season. Both are used for their health benefits.
- **Climate Considerations:** Thrives in climates with cold winters and hot summers. Avoid extremely hot or dry climates. Think of areas with distinct seasons but not harsh extremes.

How to Use Elderberry

Herbal Teas or Infusions: Elderberry flowers or dried berries are soaked in hot water to make a soothing tea known for boosting the immune system.

Tinctures: Berries or flowers are soaked in alcohol to extract the medicinal properties, used to treat colds and flu.

Salves-Topical Applications: A cream made from elderberry extract can be applied to the skin to alleviate inflammation and promote healing.

Compresses: Soaked cloth in elderberry tea or tincture can be applied to the skin to reduce swelling or pain.

Herbal Baths: Adding elderberry infusion to bath water can soothe skin irritations and promote relaxation.

Steam Inhalation: Inhaling steam from boiled elderberries or flowers can relieve respiratory congestion.

Decoctions: Boiling the roots or bark of elderberry creates a strong decoction used traditionally for kidney and bladder issues.

Syrups: Elderberry syrup, made from the juice of the berries and other ingredients, is popular for its antiviral properties and ability to alleviate cold and flu symptoms.

Gargles & Mouthwashes: A gargle made from elderberry infusion can soothe a sore throat and reduce inflammation.

Powders: Dried and powdered elderberry can be used in capsules as a supplement or added to food for extra nutrients.

Juices: Fresh elderberry juice is rich in vitamins and antioxidants, often used to boost the immune system.

Culinary Uses: Elderberries are used in cooking for making jams, jellies, and pies, adding both flavor and nutritional value.

Ease to Grow: 3-5, Low Maintenance

Elderberry is fairly easy to grow, thriving in a variety of conditions and requiring minimal care once established. With its hardiness and low maintenance requirements, elderberry is a great choice for novice gardeners, providing both medicinal benefits and wildlife support.

Elecampane

Known scientifically as Inula Helenium, a perennial herb prominent in traditional medicine, particularly for treating respiratory ailments. Its tall, sunflower-like appearance and large, broad leaves make it recognizable, thriving in damp, grassy meadows. Elecampane's roots are the primary medicinal part, harvested in autumn and valued for their high inulin content, antimicrobial, and expectorant properties.

Respiratory System

Bronchial tubes: Elecampane's root extract aids in loosening phlegm and easing breathing by acting as an expectorant, reducing bronchial tube inflammation.

Digestive System

Stomach and intestines: The inulin in Elecampane supports digestive health, promoting beneficial gut bacteria growth and aiding digestion.

Immune System

Overall immunity: Elecampane has immune-enhancing properties, helping to boost the body's defense against infections.

How to Grow Elecampane

- **Selecting the Right Variety:** Elecampane has primarily one common variety used for medicinal purposes. It's best started from root cuttings or seeds. Seeds can be purchased from herbal or specialty garden stores. Root cuttings are often more reliable and quicker to establish.
- **Best Time to Plant Outdoors:** Plant in late fall or early spring. The cooler temperatures help the plant establish without the stress of summer heat.
- **Spacing Outdoor Plants:** Space plants or seeds about 2 to 3 feet apart to allow for growth and air circulation, reducing the risk of disease.

- **Container Use and Soil:** Prefers deep pots with rich, well-drained soil. Outdoor soil should be fertile with good moisture retention but not waterlogged.
- **Sunlight and Location:** Thrives in full sun to partial shade. If using artificial lighting, LED grow lights can provide a good spectrum for growth.
- **Watering:** Keep soil consistently moist but not waterlogged. Water deeply once a week, more often in very hot weather.
- **Feeding:** Feed with a balanced liquid fertilizer monthly during the growing season to support robust growth.
- **Pruning and Maintenance:** Snip off dead flowers to encourage more blooms. Remove dead or yellowing leaves to maintain plant health.
- **Pest and Disease Management:** Watch for slug and snail damage. Rust and powdery mildew can occur; treat with appropriate fungicides and improve air circulation.
- **Overwintering:** In colder zones, mulch around the base to protect roots from freezing. In warmer climates, normal winter care is sufficient.
- **Propagation:** Propagate by dividing the roots in the fall or spring. Seed propagation is possible but less common.
- **Harvesting:** Harvest roots in the fall of the second or third year. Wash and dry them for medicinal use. Leaves and flowers can be used fresh or dried.
- **Climate Considerations:** Thrives in temperate climates. While not suited to very hot or tropical climates, it can tolerate cold well.

How to Use Elecampane

Herbal Teas or Infusions: Soak dried elecampane root in hot water for 10-15 minutes to make a tea that can help with respiratory and digestive issues.

Tinctures: The root of elecampane is often used in tincture form, extracted in alcohol, to aid in respiratory and digestive health.

Salves-Topical Applications: Infused oil from elecampane can be made into salves for skin issues and inflammation.

Decoctions: A strong decoction of elecampane root can be made for more potent therapeutic use, especially for lung health and cough relief.

Syrups: Elecampane root is commonly used in homemade cough syrups for its expectorant properties, helping to ease bronchial issues.

Powders: The dried root can be powdered and used in capsules or mixed into food or drinks for digestive support.

Culinary Uses: While not commonly used in cooking, elecampane root can be added to soups or stews for its health benefits and unique flavor.

Ease to Grow: 3-5, Low Maintenance

Elecampane is a hardy perennial that thrives in well-drained soil with full sun to partial shade. It is generally low maintenance, suitable for novice gardeners, and requires minimal care once established, making it an accessible plant for medicinal and garden use.

Eucalyptus

A genus of over 700 species of flowering trees and shrubs, most of which are native to Australia. These plants are well-known for their aromatic leaves, which are used to produce eucalyptus oil. This oil has various medicinal properties, including being an antiseptic, decongestant, and anti-inflammatory agent. Eucalyptus leaves contain compounds like eucalyptol, which have been shown to help clear respiratory tract infections, relieve pain, and reduce inflammation. The plant is also known for its fast growth and ability to adapt to a range of environments.

Respiratory System

Lungs: Eucalyptus acts as an expectorant, helping to clear mucus from the lungs and making it easier to breathe.

Bronchi: The oil from eucalyptus leaves can dilate the bronchi and bronchioles, reducing asthma symptoms and improving airflow.

Skin and Integumentary System

Skin: Eucalyptus oil has antiseptic properties that can help in healing wounds, burns, and cuts. It also has anti-inflammatory properties that can reduce skin irritation and redness.

How to Grow Eucalyptus

- **Selecting the Right Variety:** Choose a variety of eucalyptus that suits your purpose, such as Eucalyptus globulus for medicinal use or Eucalyptus Citriodora for its lemon-scented foliage. Obtain eucalyptus seeds or young plants from reputable nurseries or online suppliers specializing in native plants.
- **Best Time to Plant Outdoors:** Plant eucalyptus outdoors in spring after the last frost when the soil has warmed up.
- **Spacing Outdoor Plants:** Space eucalyptus plants at least 10-12 feet apart to allow for their rapid growth and spread.
- **Container Use and Soil:** Use well-draining soil in containers for eucalyptus, preferably a mix of potting soil and sand for good aeration.
- **Sunlight and Location:** Eucalyptus thrives in full sun, requiring at least 6-8 hours of direct sunlight per day. Indoors, provide bright light near a sunny window.
- **Watering:** Water eucalyptus regularly, keeping the soil evenly moist but not waterlogged. Allow the top inch of soil to dry between waterings.
- **Feeding:** Fertilize eucalyptus with a balanced liquid fertilizer every 4-6 weeks during the growing season to promote healthy growth.
- **Pruning and Maintenance:** Prune eucalyptus to shape it and remove dead or damaged branches. Snip off dead flowers to encourage new growth.
- **Pest and Disease Management:** Watch for pests like eucalyptus gall wasps and treat with insecticidal soap if needed. For diseases like root rot, improve drainage and avoid overwatering.

- **Overwintering:** In colder climates, protect eucalyptus from frost by wrapping young trees with burlap and mulching around the base.
- **Propagation:** Propagate eucalyptus from stem cuttings in spring or early summer for best results.
- **Harvesting:** Harvest eucalyptus leaves and twigs as needed for medicinal or aromatic purposes throughout the growing season. Avoid harvesting more than one-third of the plant at a time to ensure its continued health.
- **Climate Considerations:** Eucalyptus thrives in warm temperate climates with mild winters and hot summers, preferring a Mediterranean-like environment with well-drained soil and plenty of sunlight.

How to Use Eucalyptus

- **Herbal Teas or Infusions:** Soak eucalyptus leaves in hot water to make a soothing tea for respiratory and immune support.
- **Tinctures:** Use eucalyptus tincture for its antimicrobial properties by diluting it in water or alcohol.
- **Salves-Topical Applications:** Apply eucalyptus salves or ointments to the chest for respiratory relief or to soothe sore muscles.
- **Compresses - Aromatherapy & Essential Oils:** Inhale eucalyptus essential oil for respiratory benefits or add to a diffuser for a refreshing aroma.
- **Steam Inhalation:** Add eucalyptus oil to hot water and inhale steam to clear nasal passages and ease congestion.
- **Decoctions:** Boil eucalyptus leaves to create a strong medicinal infusion for respiratory conditions.

- **Syrups:** Make eucalyptus syrup for cough relief by combining the plant extract with honey or sugar.
- **Gargles & Mouthwashes:** Use eucalyptus gargles or mouthwashes for oral hygiene and to soothe throat irritations.
- **Powders:** Crush dried eucalyptus leaves into a powder for use in capsules or as an ingredient in herbal remedies.
- **Juices:** Extract eucalyptus juice for its medicinal properties, commonly used in traditional medicine practices.
- **Culinary Uses:** Infuse eucalyptus flavor into dishes sparingly, as it has a strong taste and may overpower other flavors.

Ease to Grow: 5-7, Medium to High Maintenance

Cultivating eucalyptus can be moderately challenging, requiring careful attention to its specific needs. While it's not overly complicated, it does demand consistent care in terms of soil, water, and sunlight to thrive successfully. With proper management and understanding of its growing requirements, eucalyptus can be grown with moderate ease, making it accessible to dedicated gardeners or herbal enthusiasts.

Fennel

A highly aromatic and flavorful herb used both as a culinary ingredient and medicinal plant. Its feathery leaves, seeds, and bulb are used in various dishes worldwide. Fennel is known for its licorice-like taste and is integral in Mediterranean cuisine. Medicinally, fennel has been used to treat a myriad of health conditions due to its potent antioxidant, anti-inflammatory, and antimicrobial properties.

Digestive System

Stomach: Fennel can alleviate stomach discomfort by reducing bloating, easing digestion, and promoting the overall health of the stomach lining.

Intestines: It helps in relaxing the muscles of the intestines, thereby reducing gas, bloating, and stomach cramps.

Respiratory System

Lungs: Fennel has expectorant properties, aiding in clearing the lungs and bronchial passages of mucus and relieving coughing.

Endocrine System

Hormonal Balance: Fennel contains compounds that mimic the estrogen hormone, which can help in balancing hormonal levels in the body.

How to Grow Fennel

- **Selecting the Right Variety:** Fennel comes in two main types: Florence fennel, which is cultivated for its bulb, and common fennel, grown for its leaves and seeds. Both types can be started from seeds, which are readily available at garden centers and online stores. Florence fennel is preferred for its edible bulb, while common fennel is known for its flavorful seeds and leaves.
- **Best Time to Plant Outdoors:** Plant fennel seeds directly in the garden in early spring, after the last frost, or in autumn in

warmer climates. Fennel prefers cooler growing conditions and can bolt (or flower early) if planted late and exposed to long days and high temperatures.

- **Spacing Outdoor Plants:** Space fennel plants 12 to 18 inches apart to allow enough room for growth. Fennel can grow quite tall, so spacing helps ensure adequate air circulation and reduces competition for nutrients.

- **Container Use and Soil:** Fennel can be grown in containers, especially the Florence variety. Use a deep pot to accommodate the plant's long taproot and well-draining soil rich in organic matter to promote healthy growth.

- **Sunlight and Location:** Fennel thrives in a sunny location, requiring at least 6 hours of direct sunlight daily. If grown indoors or in areas with less sunlight, use grow lights to supplement light exposure.

- **Watering:** Keep the soil consistently moist but not waterlogged. Fennel's deep roots require regular, deep watering to develop properly, especially during dry spells.

- **Feeding:** Apply a balanced, slow-release fertilizer at planting time and supplement with a liquid feed every few weeks to support robust growth.

- **Pruning and Maintenance:** Snip off dead flowers to prevent the plant from putting energy into seed production. Regularly check for and remove any yellowing leaves to keep the plant healthy.

- **Pest and Disease Management:** Fennel is susceptible to aphids and carrot rust flies. Regularly inspect plants and treat with organic pesticides if necessary. Ensure good air circulation and practice crop rotation to prevent fungal diseases.

- **Overwintering:** In colder climates, mulch around the base of fennel plants to protect them during winter. Florence fennel may need to be replanted annually.

- **Propagation:** Fennel can be propagated by seeds or by dividing the clumps of established plants in spring or autumn.
- **Harvesting:** Harvest fennel leaves as needed, cut bulbs when they are about the size of a tennis ball, and collect seeds once the flower heads dry and turn brown. The entire plant offers various health benefits, from the seeds to the bulb.
- **Climate Considerations:** Fennel prefers climates with sunny, mild days and cool nights. It adapts well to different environments but avoids extreme heat to prevent early flowering.

How to Use Fennel

Herbal Teas or Infusions: Fennel seeds are soaked in boiling water to make a soothing tea that aids digestion and relieves bloating.

Tinctures: Fennel seeds are steeped in alcohol to extract their essential oils, creating a concentrated tincture for digestive and respiratory issues.

Salves-Topical Applications: Crushed fennel seeds are mixed into creams or ointments for anti-inflammatory and soothing skin treatments.

Compresses: A cloth soaked in fennel tea can be applied to the skin to reduce inflammation and soothe irritations.

Aromatherapy & Essential Oils: Fennel essential oil is used in diffusers for respiratory relief and in direct skin applications for its antiseptic properties.

Herbal Baths: Fennel seeds or leaves can be added to bath water for a relaxing and skin-soothing herbal bath.

Steam Inhalation: Inhaling steam infused with fennel seeds can relieve nasal congestion and respiratory issues.

Decoctions: Fennel roots or seeds are boiled in water to make a strong decoction for treating digestive disorders.

Syrups: Fennel seed decoction is mixed with sugar to make syrups for cough and throat relief.

Gargles & Mouthwashes: A fennel infusion may be used as a gargle or mouthwash to freshen breath and treat sore throat.

Powders: Dried fennel seeds are ground into powder for use in culinary dishes or as a dietary supplement.

Juices: Fennel bulb can be juiced and consumed for its digestive and nutritional benefits.

Culinary Uses: Fennel is used extensively in cooking for its aromatic seeds and bulb, enhancing the flavor of dishes.

Ease to Grow: 2-4, Low Maintenance

Fennel is relatively easy to grow, requiring basic care like sunlight, water, and occasional feeding. It adapts well to various climates and soil types, making it a low-maintenance choice for both novice and experienced gardeners.

Fenugreek

A versatile herb with aromatic seeds and leaves used extensively in culinary and medicinal applications. It's known for its distinct maple-like flavor and health benefits. Fenugreek has been traditionally used to aid digestion, improve metabolism, and enhance lactation. Its seeds contain fibers and compounds that can help regulate blood sugar levels, making it popular for diabetes management. Fenugreek also has anti-inflammatory and antioxidant properties, contributing to its therapeutic use in treating skin conditions and soothing mucous membranes.

Digestive System

Stomach: Fenugreek aids in the production of gastric juices, helping to soothe digestive inflammation and improve digestion.

Respiratory System

Lungs: The seeds act as an expectorant, helping to alleviate congestion and reduce the severity of colds and sinus problems.

Reproductive System

Hormonal Balance: Fenugreek seeds contain phytoestrogens, contributing to a balance in hormonal levels, especially in women.

Endocrine System

Pancreas: Enhances insulin production and sensitivity, aiding in blood sugar regulation for diabetic patients.

How to Grow Fenugreek

- **Selecting the Right Variety:** Fenugreek is primarily grown from seeds. There are no specific varieties, as the standard fenugreek seed is used for both culinary and medicinal purposes. Seeds can be purchased online or at specialty gardening stores. Starting with organic, non-GMO seeds is often recommended to ensure purity and health benefits.

- **Best Time to Plant Outdoors:** Plant fenugreek seeds in spring, after the last frost, when the soil is warm. In warmer climates, it can also be planted in autumn.
- **Spacing Outdoor Plants:** Sow seeds about 1/4 inch deep and space them 2 to 3 inches apart. Rows should be spaced 6 to 18 inches apart to allow room for growth.
- **Container Use and Soil:** Fenugreek grows well in containers. Use a well-draining potting mix and ensure the container has adequate drainage holes. The plant prefers neutral to slightly acidic soil.
- **Sunlight and Location:** Fenugreek requires full sun, at least 4 to 6 hours of direct sunlight per day. If growing indoors, place it in a sunny spot or use artificial grow lights to supplement light.
- **Watering:** Keep the soil moist but not waterlogged. Water regularly, especially during dry periods, to maintain even soil moisture.
- **Feeding:** Fenugreek does not require heavy fertilization. Apply a balanced, organic fertilizer at planting time and sparingly throughout the growing season if necessary.
- **Pruning and Maintenance:** Regularly check for and remove any yellowing leaves or signs of disease. Snip off dead flowers to prevent the plant from flowering too early and focus its energy on leaf production.
- **Pest and Disease Management:** Watch for common pests like aphids. Diseases such as powdery mildew can occur; treat with organic fungicides and ensure good air circulation around plants.
- **Overwintering:** Fenugreek is generally grown as an annual, so overwintering is not typically necessary. In mild climates, it may survive winter and regrow in spring.

- **Propagation:** Propagate fenugreek by seed. It doesn't transplant well, so it's best to sow directly in the final growing spot.
- **Harvesting:** Leaves can be harvested once they are large enough to use, typically 3 to 4 weeks after sowing. Seeds are ready when the pods are yellow and the seeds within make a rattling sound when shaken; this usually occurs 3 to 4 months after planting.
- **Climate Considerations:** Fenugreek thrives in warm and sunny conditions. While it can grow in various climates, it does best in areas with hot summers and mild winters, avoiding extreme cold or frost.

How to Use Fenugreek

Herbal Teas or Infusions: Fenugreek seeds are soaked in hot water to make herbal tea, which is consumed for its health benefits, especially to aid digestion and lactation.

Tinctures: The seeds are soaked in alcohol to extract their beneficial compounds, creating a concentrated liquid used medicinally.

Salves-Topical Applications: Ground fenugreek seeds are mixed with oils to make creams or ointments for skin inflammation and wounds.

Poultices: Crushed fenugreek leaves or seeds are mixed with water to form a paste, applied to the skin to reduce inflammation and pain.

Compresses: A cloth soaked in fenugreek-infused water can be applied to the skin to soothe inflammation and skin issues.

Decoctions: Fenugreek seeds are boiled in water for a long time to make a decoction, which can be used to treat respiratory conditions.

Syrups: The extract from fenugreek seeds is mixed with sweeteners to make a syrup, often used to ease cough and sore throat.

Powders: Dried fenugreek leaves or seeds are ground into powder, used for culinary purposes, and as a dietary supplement.

Culinary Uses: Fenugreek seeds and leaves are used in cooking, especially in Indian cuisine, for their distinctive flavor and health benefits.

Ease to Grow: 2-4, Low Maintenance

Fenugreek is relatively easy to grow, requiring minimal care. It thrives in warm climates and well-drained soil. Regular watering and occasional feeding will support healthy growth. It's a robust plant, resistant to many pests and diseases, making it a good choice for beginners in gardening.

Feverfew

Perennial herb with daisy-like flowers, has been used for centuries in traditional medicine, particularly for treating headaches, migraines, and fevers. Its active compounds, including parthenolide, have anti-inflammatory and pain-relieving properties. Feverfew is often explored for its potential in treating arthritis and rheumatic diseases. Its leaves are commonly consumed fresh or dried, and are available in various forms like capsules, tablets, and tinctures.

Nervous System

Headaches and Migraines: Feverfew reduces the frequency and severity of migraines by inhibiting serotonin release and reducing inflammation in blood vessels.

Cardiovascular System

Blood Vessels: Feverfew aids in maintaining cardiovascular health by preventing the constriction of blood vessels, thus improving blood flow and reducing the risk of clots.

Immune System

Inflammatory Response: Feverfew modulates the immune system by inhibiting the release of inflammatory substances, which can help in reducing chronic inflammation and supporting overall immune health.

How to Grow Feverfew

- **Selecting the Right Variety:** Feverfew is available in various cultivars. The most common type is Tanacetum Parthenium. It's generally grown from seeds, which can be purchased online or at garden centers. Some prefer planting seedlings for a head start.
- **Best Time to Plant Outdoors:** Plant Feverfew seeds or starts in early spring after the last frost. The plant tolerates a range of conditions but prefers cooler temperatures.
- **Spacing Outdoor Plants:** Space plants or seeds about 12 to 18 inches apart to allow for growth and airflow, reducing the risk of disease.
- **Container Use and Soil:** Feverfew thrives in well-drained soil and can be grown in containers. Use a standard potting mix and ensure pots have drainage holes.

- **Sunlight and Location:** Prefers full sun to partial shade, needing around 4-6 hours of sunlight daily. If using artificial lighting, fluorescent grow lights are suitable.
- **Watering:** Water regularly to keep the soil moist but not waterlogged. Reduce watering frequency once plants are established.
- **Feeding:** Apply a balanced liquid fertilizer monthly during the growing season to support healthy growth.
- **Pruning and Maintenance:** Regularly snip off dead flowers to encourage more blooms. This prevents the plant from flowering too early and promotes foliage growth.
- **Pest and Disease Management:** Watch for aphids and spider mites. Treat infestations with insecticidal soap. Prevent fungal diseases by ensuring good air circulation and not overcrowding plants.
- **Overwintering:** In colder climates, mulch around the base to protect roots from freezing temperatures.
- **Propagation:** Easily propagated by seed in spring or by division in autumn. Seedlings can self-sow extensively.
- **Harvesting:** Leaves can be picked any time during the growing season. Harvest leaves in the morning when the concentration of active compounds is highest.
- **Climate Considerations:** Thrives in temperate climates but can adapt to various environmental conditions. Avoid excessively hot and dry climates.

How to Use Feverfew

Herbal Teas or Infusions: Soak feverfew leaves in hot water to make a tea. It is used to reduce fever and alleviate headaches.

Tinctures: Fresh or dried feverfew leaves are soaked in alcohol to extract the active ingredients, creating a tincture that is used for migraine prevention.

Salves-Topical Applications: Feverfew is infused into a cream or ointment and applied topically to ease joint pains and skin irritation.

Decoctions: Boiled feverfew leaves create a strong liquid used to ease digestive issues and improve appetite.

Gargles & Mouthwashes: A decoction of feverfew is cooled and used as a gargle or mouthwash to relieve mouth ulcers and sore throats.

Powders: Dried and powdered feverfew leaves are used in capsules or mixed with creams for anti-inflammatory and analgesic effects.

Culinary Uses: Although not commonly used in cooking, young feverfew leaves can be added in small amounts to salads for a bitter flavor.

Ease to Grow: 2-4, Low Maintenance

Feverfew is a hardy, low-maintenance plant that grows easily in a range of conditions. It prefers full sun but tolerates partial shade and is not fussy about soil type, making it suitable for novice gardeners. Its resilience and self-seeding nature make it an easy addition to many gardens.

Garlic

Known scientifically as Allium Sativum, a plant with a long history of use both as a food and a medicine. Cultivated worldwide, it's recognized for its strong aroma and flavor, enhancing numerous culinary dishes. Beyond its culinary uses, garlic has been traditionally used to treat various health issues. Its health benefits are attributed to its compound allicin and other sulfur-containing compounds, antioxidants, and anti-inflammatory properties.

Cardiovascular System

Blood Pressure: Garlic helps lower blood pressure by dilating blood vessels, improving blood flow, and reducing arterial pressure.

Cholesterol Levels: Regular consumption of garlic can reduce both total cholesterol and LDL cholesterol levels, contributing to heart health.

Immune System

Immune Enhancement: Garlic boosts immune function by increasing the activity of immune cells like macrophages and lymphocytes, enhancing the body's ability to fight infections.

Antioxidant Protection: The antioxidants in garlic help protect immune cells from damage and support overall immune health.

Digestive System

Gastrointestinal Health: Garlic stimulates digestion and appetite, aids in detoxifying the body, and supports the health of the gastrointestinal tract.

Respiratory System

Lung Health: Garlic has been used to clear respiratory tract infections, acting as an expectorant to relieve congestion in the lungs.

How to Grow Garlic

- **Selecting the Right Variety:** Garlic varieties include Softneck, Hardneck, and Black Garlic. Softneck is common and stores well, Hardneck offers rich flavor, and Black Garlic, aged under controlled conditions, has a sweet taste. Prefer starting with cloves rather than seeds. Purchase from garden centers, nurseries, or online stores.
- **Best Time to Plant Outdoors:** Plant garlic in the fall, about 4-6 weeks before the ground freezes, to allow for root establishment without sprouting.
- **Spacing Outdoor Plants:** Plant cloves 4 to 6 inches apart in rows spaced 1 to 2 feet apart to ensure adequate room for growth.
- **Container Use and Soil:** Garlic can grow in containers; use well-draining soil rich in organic matter. Outdoor soil should be loose, fertile, and well-drained.
- **Sunlight and Location:** Garlic requires full sun, needing 6-8 hours of direct sunlight daily. In regions with hot climates, some shade is beneficial.
- **Watering:** Keep the soil evenly moist. Water when the top inch of soil feels dry, especially during bulb formation.
- **Feeding:** Apply a balanced, slow-release fertilizer at planting and an additional nitrogen boost in the spring.
- **Pruning and Maintenance:** Remove any flowers early to ensure energy is directed towards bulb growth, not seed production.
- **Pest and Disease Management:** Watch for signs of rust, white rot, and onion maggot. Rotate crops and use organic fungicides or pesticides as needed.
- **Overwintering:** In colder zones, mulch with straw or leaves to protect the cloves during winter.

- **Propagation:** Garlic is propagated through planting individual cloves from a bulb.
- **Harvesting:** Harvest garlic when the lower leaves turn brown but the upper leaves are still green. Carefully dig up the bulbs, shake off the soil, and let them cure in a dry, ventilated area.
- **Climate Considerations:** Garlic thrives in a climate with a cold winter and a warm, dry summer. It's less suitable for very wet or tropical climates.

How to Use Garlic

Herbal Teas or Infusions: Garlic cloves are soaked in hot water to create an infusion known for its health benefits, particularly for colds and flu.

Tinctures: Garlic is macerated in alcohol to produce a tincture, used for its antimicrobial properties.

Salves-Topical Applications: Crushed garlic is mixed into creams or ointments for treating fungal infections and wounds.

Compresses: A cloth soaked in garlic-infused water is applied to the skin to alleviate inflammation and infection.

Decoctions: Boiling garlic in water makes a strong decoction used for respiratory and digestive issues.

Syrups: Garlic syrup, made by simmering garlic in water and adding honey, is used to relieve coughs and sore throats.

Gargles & Mouthwashes: A solution made from garlic steeped in water can be used as a gargle or mouthwash to treat oral infections.

Culinary Uses: Garlic is widely used in cooking for flavoring dishes; along with its massive nutritional and medicinal benefits.

Ease to Grow: 2-4, Low Maintenance

Garlic is relatively easy to grow, thriving in diverse climates with minimal care. It requires good soil, adequate sunlight, and regular watering. Harvesting involves simple steps of pulling bulbs from the soil, making it accessible for gardeners of all skill levels.

Ginger

Scientifically known as Zingiber Officinale, is a flowering plant whose rhizome, ginger root, is widely used as a spice and folk medicine. Originating from Southeast Asia, it's now cultivated worldwide for its culinary and therapeutic properties. Ginger's signature aroma and flavor come from its natural oils, the most important of which is gingerol.

Digestive System

Stomach: Ginger helps alleviate nausea and vomiting, promoting gastric emptying and stimulating antral contractions.

Intestines: Aids in reducing intestinal gas and bloating by enhancing digestive activity and saliva flow.

Respiratory System

Lungs: Ginger acts as an expectorant, helping to clear mucus from the lungs and soothing respiratory pathways.

Cardiovascular System

Blood Circulation: Ginger improves blood circulation by dilating blood vessels and has a warming effect on the body.

Cholesterol Levels: It can help reduce cholesterol levels, thereby decreasing the risk of heart disease.

Immune System

Immune Response: Ginger boosts the immune system by stimulating the body's natural defense mechanisms against infections and diseases.

Muscular System

Ginger's anti-inflammatory properties are beneficial in relieving muscle pain and soreness, often used to soothe post-exercise inflammation.

How to Grow Ginger

- **Selecting the Right Variety:** Ginger varieties like Maran, Athira, and Varada are popular due to their high yield and quality. It's preferable to start with fresh rhizomes rather than seeds or starts. You can purchase these from nurseries, online garden stores, or local farmers' markets.
- **Best Time to Plant Outdoors:** Plant ginger in late winter or early spring, after the last frost, when the soil is warm.
- **Spacing Outdoor Plants:** Plant ginger rhizomes about 8 inches apart in rows that are spaced 1 to 2 feet apart to allow for growth and airflow.
- **Container Use and Soil:** Ginger thrives in large pots with well-draining, fertile soil rich in organic matter. Use a mix of garden soil, compost, and perlite or sand for good drainage.
- **Sunlight and Location:** Ginger prefers partial shade with 2-5 hours of direct sunlight per day. In hotter climates, indirect

sunlight is better. For artificial lighting, use grow lights positioned 12-18 inches above the plants.

- **Watering:** Keep the soil consistently moist but not waterlogged. Water ginger plants deeply once a week, more often in hot, dry weather.
- **Feeding:** Apply a balanced, slow-release fertilizer every 4-6 weeks during the growing season to support growth.
- **Pruning and Maintenance:** Snip off any dead flowers or yellow leaves to encourage growth. Regularly check for pests and diseases and act promptly to mitigate any issues.
- **Pest and Disease Management:** Watch for common issues like ginger rhizome rot and leaf spot. Keep plants healthy to avoid pests, and use organic fungicides or neem oil for treatment.
- **Overwintering:** In cooler climates, mulch ginger beds with straw or bring containers indoors to protect from frost.
- **Propagation:** Divide ginger rhizomes with a few growth buds each and replant to propagate new plants.
- **Harvesting:** Harvest ginger when the leaves turn yellow and dry, typically 8-10 months after planting. Carefully dig up the rhizomes, which can be used fresh, dried, or powdered.
- **Climate Considerations:** Ginger grows best in warm, humid climates with consistent temperatures between 75-85°F. Avoid areas with heavy frost or very high heat.

How to Use Ginger

Herbal Teas or Infusions: Ginger can be soaked in boiling water for 10-15 minutes to make a spicy, warming tea. Also aids in digestion and relieves nausea.

Tinctures: Ginger tincture is made by soaking the root in alcohol, which extracts its active compounds, used for digestive issues and inflammation.

Salves-Topical Applications: Ginger is used in creams for its anti-inflammatory properties, helping to relieve pain and swelling in conditions like arthritis.

Decoctions: Boiling ginger root in water makes a strong decoction, useful for treating colds and respiratory issues.

Syrups: Ginger syrup, made from the root's extract and sugar, soothes sore throats and coughs.

Culinary Uses: Fresh, dried, or powdered ginger is used in cooking for its flavor and as a digestive aid.

Ease to Grow: 2-4, Low Maintenance

Ginger is relatively easy to grow, thriving in warm, humid environments and requiring minimal maintenance. It's grown from rhizomes, which can be planted in well-draining soil and kept moist.

Ginkgo Biloba

Often simply called ginkgo, is a living fossil with no known living relatives and is known for its distinctive fan-shaped leaves. Originating in China, ginkgo has been cultivated for millennia for its aesthetic and medicinal properties. It is revered for its robustness and longevity, with some specimens living over a thousand years. In traditional medicine, ginkgo leaves are used to enhance cognitive function and improve memory and concentration. The plant's therapeutic properties are attributed to its high content of flavonoids and terpenoids, which have antioxidant and anti-inflammatory effects.

Nervous System

Cognitive Function: Ginkgo Biloba enhances cognitive function by improving blood flow to the brain and protecting nerve cells.

Memory Enhancement: It is reputed to boost memory and cognitive speed, which is especially beneficial in age-related cognitive decline.

Cardiovascular System

Blood Circulation: Ginkgo Biloba improves blood circulation by dilating blood vessels and reducing blood viscosity.

Vascular Health: It supports vascular health by maintaining the elasticity and tone of blood vessels, helping to prevent arteriosclerosis (hardening of the arteries).

Respiratory System

Lung Function: Ginkgo helps in improving lung function and has been used to treat conditions like asthma by reducing inflammation in the respiratory tract.

How to Grow Ginkgo Biloba

- **Selecting the Right Variety:** Ginkgo Biloba has several cultivars, but 'Autumn Gold' and 'Saratoga' are popular for their growth habits and leaf shape. Starting with seeds is possible but slow; nursery-bought saplings are more common. Ginkgo trees are available at nurseries and online garden centers, ensuring a better start than growing from seed due to the long germination period.

- **Best Time to Plant Outdoors:** The ideal planting time is during the spring or fall when the weather is mild. This timing allows the roots to establish before extreme temperatures in summer or winter.

- **Spacing Outdoor Plants:** Plant ginkgo trees at least 20 feet apart to accommodate their mature size and ensure proper air circulation.

- **Container Use and Soil:** While young ginkgo can be grown in pots, they eventually need to be planted in the ground. Use well-draining soil, rich in organic matter, for both container and ground planting.

- **Sunlight and Location:** Ginkgo prefers full sun to partial shade, requiring at least 4-6 hours of direct sunlight daily. If using artificial lighting, LED grow lights that mimic natural sunlight can be used for young plants indoors.

- **Watering:** Water young trees regularly to keep the soil moist but not waterlogged. Once established, ginkgo trees are drought-tolerant and require less frequent watering.

- **Feeding:** Apply a balanced, slow-release fertilizer in early spring to support growth.

- **Pruning and Maintenance:** Minimal pruning is needed. Remove any dead or damaged branches and periodically check for signs of disease or pests. Snip off dead flowers to prevent unwanted seedlings.

- **Pest and Disease Management:** Ginkgo trees are remarkably resistant to pests and diseases. Monitor for signs like discolored leaves or damaged bark and consult a horticulturist if unusual symptoms appear.

- **Overwintering:** Ginkgo trees are cold-hardy and do not require special care in winter once established.

- **Propagation:** Propagation is usually done through seeds or grafting, but it requires patience as ginkgo trees grow slowly.
- **Harvesting:** Leaves are the primary harvestable part, collected in late summer or early autumn. They are used for medicinal purposes, such as making extracts or teas.
- **Climate Considerations:** Ginkgo Biloba thrives in temperate climates with distinct seasons but can adapt to a wide range of conditions. It is frost-tolerant and can grow in areas with cold winters and hot summers.

How to Use Ginkgo Biloba

Herbal Teas or Infusions: Ginkgo leaves are soaked in hot water for several minutes to make herbal tea. This infusion is consumed to potentially enhance cognitive function and improve memory.

Tinctures: Leaves of Ginkgo Biloba are soaked in alcohol to extract active compounds, creating a tincture. This tincture is used to promote blood circulation and cognitive health.

Decoctions: Ginkgo leaves are boiled in water for a long time to make a strong decoction. This liquid is taken to harness the anti-inflammatory and antioxidant properties of the plant.

Powders: Dried ginkgo leaves are ground into a fine powder, which can be used as a dietary supplement or added to smoothies and other foods for its potential health benefits.

Culinary Uses: Though not as common, ginkgo seeds (nuts) are used in Asian cuisine, particularly in soups and with other dishes, but they should be consumed in moderation due to potential toxins.

Ease to Grow: 4-6, Medium Maintenance

Ginkgo Biloba is a hardy tree once established, but it grows slowly and requires patience. It can adapt to various soil types and environmental conditions, although it does best with consistent watering and sunny locations. It's relatively easy to care for, making it medium maintenance.

Ginseng

A revered herb in traditional medicine, has been used for centuries, particularly in East Asia. Known scientifically as Panax Ginseng, it is prized for its thick, forked root which contains active compounds known as ginsenosides. These compounds are thought to be responsible for the plant's medicinal properties. Ginseng is often consumed to enhance overall health and stamina, and is believed to support various bodily functions and systems. Its reputation as a tonic for vitality and its use in various herbal remedies underline its importance in herbal medicine.

Nervous System

Brain: Ginseng may enhance cognitive functions, improving memory, concentration, and mood.

Cardiovascular System

Blood vessels: Ginseng is known to promote heart health by improving blood circulation and reducing inflammation.
Heart: It may also help in strengthening the heart muscle and improving its overall functionality.

Immune System

General immunity: Ginseng can boost the immune system, enhancing the body's resistance to illness and infection.

Endocrine System

Pancreas: Ginseng may aid in regulating blood sugar levels, which is beneficial for pancreatic health.

Adrenal glands: It is known to help in regulating the body's hormonal response to stress.

How to Grow Ginseng

- **Selecting the Right Variety:** Ginseng varieties include Asian ginseng (Panax ginseng) and American ginseng (Panax Quinquefolius). Both are valued for their medicinal properties. It's often preferable to start with stratified seeds or seedlings rather than full-grown plants. These can be purchased from reputable nurseries or online suppliers specializing in medicinal herbs.
- **Best Time to Plant Outdoors:** Plant ginseng in the fall, allowing the seeds to take hold naturally through the winter for spring germination.
- **Spacing Outdoor Plants:** Space plants or seeds about 8 to 10 inches apart to allow enough room for growth and root development.
- **Container Use and Soil:** Ginseng grows well in deep, well-drained pots with a mix of loamy and sandy soil. Ensure the container has good drainage.
- **Sunlight and Location:** Ginseng prefers 75% to 80% shade, thriving under a canopy of trees or shade cloth. If using artificial light, mimic natural conditions with low, indirect lighting.

- **Watering:** Keep the soil moist but not waterlogged. Water regularly, especially during dry spells, to maintain consistent soil moisture.
- **Feeding:** Apply a balanced, slow-release fertilizer at the beginning of the growing season to support growth without overstimulating.
- **Pruning and Maintenance:** Snip off dead flowers to promote healthy plant growth and prevent energy wastage.
- **Pest and Disease Management:** Watch for signs of root rot or fungal diseases, indicated by wilting or discolored leaves. Use organic fungicides and ensure proper soil drainage to combat these issues.
- **Overwintering:** In colder climates, mulch heavily around the plants to protect the roots from freezing temperatures.
- **Propagation:** Propagate ginseng through seed planting or by dividing older plants in the fall, ensuring each section has at least one bud.
- **Harvesting:** The roots of ginseng, its most valuable part, can be harvested after 5 to 6 years when they have accumulated significant ginsenosides (natural compounds). Dig carefully to avoid damaging the root, which can be used fresh or dried for medicinal purposes.
- **Climate Considerations:** Ginseng thrives in cool to temperate climates with high humidity and prefers a forest-like environment with shaded areas.

How to Use Ginseng

Herbal Teas or Infusions: Ginseng root can be sliced and soaked in hot water for several minutes to make a revitalizing tea that supports overall health and energy.

Tinctures: The root is often soaked in alcohol to extract its active compounds, creating a concentrated tincture that can be taken in small doses.

Salves-Topical Applications: Ginseng can be incorporated into creams or ointments for topical application to help soothe skin irritations and improve skin health.

Decoctions: A strong decoction can be made by simmering ginseng root in water for a longer period, concentrating its beneficial properties for digestive and immune support.

Syrups: Ginseng root can be added to syrups, often combined with other herbs, to create a pleasant-tasting remedy for coughs and respiratory health.

Powders: Dried ginseng can be ground into a powder and used in capsules or mixed into food or smoothies for an easy way to consume its benefits.

Ease to Grow: 5-7, Medium Maintenance

Ginseng requires careful attention to soil conditions, shade, and moisture, making it moderately challenging to cultivate. It thrives in well-drained, forest-like environments with consistent moisture and shade.

Goldenseal

(Hydrastis Canadensis) is a perennial herb native to North America, recognized by its small, greenish-white flowers and red berries. It's highly valued in herbal medicine, primarily for its root and rhizome, which contain alkaloids like berberine. Traditionally used by Native Americans, goldenseal has become popular worldwide for its therapeutic properties. It thrives in shaded, wooded areas, reflecting its preference for rich, well-drained soil and partial sunlight. Overharvesting and habitat loss have led to its status as an endangered species in the wild.

Digestive System
Mucous Membranes: Goldenseal acts on the mucous membranes, helping to reduce inflammation and treat gastrointestinal infections.

Respiratory System
Nasal Passages: Goldenseal is used to treat nasal congestion and inflammation, working as an antimicrobial agent against the pathogens causing sinusitis.

Immune System
Immune Response: Enhances the immune response by increasing

the activity of macrophages, which destroy bacteria and other pathogens.

Skin and Integumentary System

Skin Infections: Goldenseal is beneficial for treating skin infections; and has antimicrobial properties that help to fight bacteria and fungi on the skin.

How to Grow Goldenseal

- **Selecting the Right Variety:** Goldenseal typically does not have distinct varieties in the commercial sense. It is crucial to obtain healthy, disease-free roots or rhizomes (underground stems) for planting. You can purchase these from reputable nurseries or specialty herb suppliers. Ensure the plant material is ethically sourced to avoid contributing to the overharvesting of wild populations.

- **Best Time to Plant Outdoors:** Plant goldenseal in the fall or early spring when the weather is cool. This timing allows the plants to establish roots before extreme temperatures in summer or winter.

- **Spacing Outdoor Plants:** Space plants about 8 to 12 inches apart to ensure enough room for growth. This spacing helps prevent overcrowding and promotes better air circulation, reducing the risk of disease.

- **Container Use and Soil:** Goldenseal thrives in well-draining, rich, loamy soil with a high organic matter content. If growing in containers, ensure the pot has good drainage holes and use a soil mix designed for woodland plants.

- **Sunlight and Location:** Goldenseal prefers partial shade, mimicking its natural woodland habitat. Aim for a location that receives filtered sunlight or 2 to 4 hours of direct sun daily.

For artificial lighting, use grow lights that mimic the spectral output of natural sunlight.

- **Watering:** Keep the soil consistently moist but not waterlogged. Water when the top inch of soil feels dry to the touch to avoid overwatering, which leads to root rot.

- **Feeding:** Apply a balanced, slow-release organic fertilizer at the beginning of the growing season to support healthy growth. Over-fertilizing can harm the plant, so follow the recommended rates.

- **Pruning and Maintenance:** Regularly remove dead or yellowing leaves to encourage healthy growth. Snip off dead flowers to prevent the plant from flowering too early and focus energy on root development.

- **Pest and Disease Management:** Watch for signs of fungal diseases like root rot, which manifests as wilting and yellowing leaves. Improve air circulation and reduce soil moisture to manage these issues. Use organic fungicides if necessary.

- **Overwintering:** In colder climates, mulch around the base of the plants to protect the roots from freezing temperatures. Remove the mulch in spring to allow new growth.

- **Propagation:** Propagate goldenseal by dividing the rhizomes in early spring or fall. Each division should have at least one bud or eye to develop into a new plant.

- **Harvesting:** Harvest goldenseal roots after the plant is well established, typically in the third or fourth year. Dig up the roots in autumn, carefully clean them, and dry them for medicinal use. The roots and rhizomes are the most commonly used parts for their therapeutic properties.

- **Climate Considerations:** Goldenseal grows best in climates that have cold winters and mild summers. It prefers regions with consistent moisture and well-drained soil, avoiding extremely hot or arid environments.

How to Use Goldenseal

Herbal Teas or Infusions: Goldenseal leaves or roots are soaked in hot water for several minutes to create a potent herbal tea, often used to support digestive and immune system health.

Tinctures: A liquid extract of goldenseal root, often mixed with alcohol, is used as a tincture to take advantage of its medicinal properties, especially for immune support and as an antimicrobial agent.

Salves-Topical Applications: Goldenseal is incorporated into creams, ointments, or poultices for its antiseptic and healing properties, applied directly to skin irritations, wounds, or infections.

Decoctions: The root is boiled in water for a period to make a decoction, concentrating its active compounds, used to soothe sore throats or digestive issues when cooled and consumed.

Gargles & Mouthwashes: A decoction of goldenseal is often used as a gargle or mouthwash to help treat mouth ulcers, sore throats, or gum diseases due to its antimicrobial and anti-inflammatory properties.

Powders: Dried goldenseal root is ground into a powder, which can be used to sprinkle on wounds for its antimicrobial and healing benefits or ingested in capsule form for internal health benefits.

Ease to Grow: 4-6, Medium Maintenance

Goldenseal is moderately challenging to cultivate, requiring specific soil conditions and shade. It prefers a wooded environment with rich, well-draining soil. It's sensitive to overwatering and does require a bit of horticultural knowledge to manage its needs effectively, especially to grow successfully in non-native environments.

Gotu Kola

Scientifically Centella Asiatica, is a perennial herb native to the wetlands of Asia. Renowned for its medicinal properties, Gotu Kola has been used in traditional medicine for centuries. The plant's leaves and stems are rich in compounds that contribute to its therapeutic effects. Gotu Kola is not just a culinary herb but also a staple in herbal medicine, known for its ability to enhance cognitive function, heal skin issues, and improve circulation. It thrives in and around water, making it a common sight in marshy areas.

Nervous System

Neurons: Contains compounds that support neuron health, enhancing memory, focus, and cognitive function.

Skin and Integumentary System

Skin Cells: Promotes collagen production, aiding in wound healing, and reducing scars and stretch marks.

Cardiovascular System

Blood Vessels: Gotu Kola strengthens the vascular system, improving blood circulation and the integrity of veins and capillaries.

How to Grow Gotu Kola

- **Selecting the Right Variety:** Gotu Kola, or Centella Asiatica, doesn't have widely recognized varieties for medicinal use; most share similar properties. It's generally propagated from cuttings rather than seeds for quicker, more reliable results. You can purchase plants or cuttings from herbal nurseries or online stores specializing in medicinal herbs. Seeds are available but can be challenging to germinate.
- **Best Time to Plant Outdoors:** Plant in early spring after the last frost. Gotu Kola thrives in warm, moist conditions and will grow throughout the summer.
- **Spacing Outdoor Plants:** Space plants or seeds about 6 to 12 inches apart to allow for sprawling growth.
- **Container Use and Soil:** Prefers containers with rich, well-draining soil, high in organic matter. Ideal for indoor growth if outdoor conditions are too harsh.
- **Sunlight and Location:** Gotu Kola prefers partial shade but can tolerate full sun in cooler climates. Aim for at least 4-6 hours of sunlight daily. In very hot climates, protect from afternoon sun.
- **Watering:** Keep the soil consistently moist but not waterlogged. Gotu Kola enjoys wet conditions, mimicking its natural swampy habitat.
- **Feeding:** Fertilize lightly with a balanced organic fertilizer; it doesn't require heavy feeding.
- **Pruning and Maintenance:** Regularly snip off dead flowers or leaves to encourage bushier growth. The plant is low maintenance and doesn't typically need pruning.
- **Pest and Disease Management:** Watch for slugs and snails, which are common pests. Fungal diseases can occur in overly

wet conditions; ensure good air circulation and drainage to prevent issues.

- **Overwintering:** In cooler climates, mulch heavily or bring containers indoors to protect from frost.
- **Propagation:** Propagate by dividing the roots in spring or autumn, or take stem cuttings in summer.
- **Harvesting:** Harvest leaves throughout the growing season; they can be used fresh or dried for later use. Pick leaves in the morning after dew has evaporated for best potency.
- **Climate Considerations:** Thrives in warm, humid climates similar to its native tropical environment. In cooler areas, it needs protection from frost and prefers a greenhouse or indoor setting with humidity control.

How to Use Gotu Kola

Herbal Teas or Infusions: Soak Gotu Kola leaves in hot water for 5-10 minutes to make a soothing tea, which is good for enhancing memory and improving circulation.

Tinctures: Fresh or dried Gotu Kola leaves are soaked in alcohol to extract their active compounds, creating a concentrated tincture that supports mental clarity and skin health.

Salves-Topical Applications: Often used in creams or ointments for its wound-healing properties. It's applied directly to the skin to reduce scarring and improve skin elasticity.

Decoctions: Boil Gotu Kola leaves for a longer period to make a strong decoction, which can be used to aid digestion and promote liver health.

Powders: Dried Gotu Kola leaves are ground into a powder and consumed in capsules or mixed with water, beneficial for cognitive function and as a general tonic.

Culinary Uses: Fresh Gotu Kola leaves are added to salads and dishes for their health benefits, including detoxifying the body and enhancing brain function.

Ease to Grow: 3-5, Low Maintenance

Gotu Kola is a low-maintenance plant that adapts well to various conditions, thriving in partial shade and moist soil. It's easily propagated from cuttings or seeds, making it accessible for gardeners of all skill levels.

Hawthorn

A plant known for its small, sharp thorns and red berries. It is commonly found in Europe, North America, and Asia. Hawthorn has been used for centuries in traditional medicine to treat various ailments, particularly those related to the heart and blood vessels. The plant is rich in bioflavonoids, which are antioxidants that help to improve blood flow and stabilize blood vessel walls. It's also known for its sedative properties, aiding in sleep and reducing anxiety.

Cardiovascular System

Heart muscle: Hawthorn strengthens cardiac output by increasing the force of heart contractions and improving coronary artery blood flow.

Blood vessels: It helps in dilating blood vessels, improving blood flow, and reducing blood pressure.

Digestive System

Digestive tract: Hawthorn has been used to aid digestion and improve the breakdown of fatty foods.

Nervous System

Stress response: By reducing blood pressure and having a calming effect, Hawthorn may help alleviate stress and reduce anxiety symptoms.

How to Grow Hawthorn

- **Selecting the Right Variety:** Hawthorn comes in several species with Crataegus Monogyna and Crataegus Laevigata being the most common. Choose based on the size and type of fruit or flower desired. It is generally preferable to start with seedlings or young plants, which can be purchased from nurseries or garden centers.
- **Best Time to Plant Outdoors:** Plant hawthorn in late fall or early spring when the weather is cool. This timing helps the plant to establish roots without the stress of extreme heat or cold.
- **Spacing Outdoor Plants:** Space hawthorn trees 15 to 20 feet apart to allow for mature growth and adequate air circulation.
- **Container Use and Soil:** Hawthorn can grow in a large container with well-draining soil. It prefers loamy soil with a mix of clay, sand, and organic matter.
- **Sunlight and Location:** Plant in a location that receives at least 6 to 8 hours of direct sunlight daily. If using artificial lighting, full-spectrum LED lights are suitable.

- **Watering:** Water young plants regularly to keep the soil moist but not waterlogged. Mature hawthorn trees are drought-tolerant but benefit from occasional watering during long dry spells.
- **Feeding:** Apply a balanced fertilizer in early spring and again in mid-summer to support healthy growth.
- **Pruning and Maintenance:** Snip off dead flowers in early spring to promote new growth. Prune to shape the tree and remove any dead or diseased branches.
- **Pest and Disease Management:** Watch for signs of rust, leaf spot, and aphids. Treat with appropriate organic or chemical solutions as needed.
- **Overwintering:** In colder climates, young plants may need mulch around the base for winter protection.
- **Propagation:** Propagate by seeds, cuttings, or layering in the autumn. Seeds require cold stratification (exposure to cold) before planting .
- **Harvesting:** Flowers and leaves can be harvested in late spring; berries are best picked when fully ripe in the fall. The plant parts are used for their medicinal properties, particularly in supporting cardiovascular health.
- **Climate Considerations:** Hawthorn thrives in temperate climates with distinct seasons. It can tolerate frost and prefers a cooler climate over hot, dry conditions. Hawthorn adapts well to areas with cold winters and moderate summers.

How to Use Hawthorn

Herbal Teas or Infusions: Soak dried hawthorn leaves and flowers in hot water for 10 to 15 minutes to make a soothing tea that supports heart health.

Tinctures: Hawthorn berries, leaves, and flowers are used to make tinctures that help improve cardiovascular function and lower blood pressure.

Salves-Topical Applications: Infused oil from hawthorn berries can be used in creams and ointments to soothe inflamed skin.

Compresses: A compress made with hawthorn tea can be applied to the skin to reduce inflammation and pain.

Decoctions: Boil hawthorn berries to create a strong decoction that can be taken to aid digestion and heart health.

Syrups: Hawthorn berry syrup is used for its expectorant properties, helping to treat respiratory conditions.

Gargles & Mouthwashes: A hawthorn infusion can be used as a gargle or mouthwash to soothe sore throats.

Culinary Uses: Hawthorn berries are edible and can be used in jellies, jams, and beverages.

Ease to Grow: 2-4, Low Maintenance

Hawthorn is a resilient plant that adapts well to various environments, making it low maintenance and easy to grow. It thrives in temperate climates with full sun to partial shade and requires minimal care once established.

Holy Basil

Also known as Tulsi, is a revered plant in traditional Ayurvedic medicine, known for its fragrant leaves and robust health benefits. It is a versatile herb that grows easily in warm climates and is used both in culinary and therapeutic contexts. Holy Basil is particularly noted for its adaptogenic properties, helping the body cope with stress and promoting mental balance.

Digestive System

Stomach: Holy Basil aids in digestion and can help to relieve stomach cramps and reduce gastric acidity.

Nervous System

Stress response: Holy Basil is known to counteract stress effects by regulating cortisol levels, thus acting as an adaptogen (helper to relieve stress).

Respiratory System

Lungs: Supports respiratory health by helping to clear congestion and relieve symptoms of colds, flu, and bronchitis.

Cardiovascular System

Blood vessels: Holy Basil can contribute to cardiovascular health by helping to maintain normal blood pressure levels and supporting heart function.

Immune System

General immunity: Enhances immune response by increasing the activity of immune cells and reducing inflammation. Also enhances immune response, with its anti-inflammatory and antimicrobial properties, helping to ward off infections.

Endocrine System

Pancreas: It may help in regulating blood sugar levels, thus supporting pancreatic function and aiding in diabetes management.

How to Grow Holy Basil

- **Selecting the Right Variety:** Holy Basil, or Tulsi, comes in several varieties, including Rama Tulsi, Krishna Tulsi, and Vana Tulsi. Rama Tulsi has light green leaves and a milder flavor, Krishna Tulsi has darker leaves with a stronger aroma, and Vana Tulsi is known for its hardiness and spicy flavor. Starting from seeds is common, and they can be purchased from specialized online herb stores or local nurseries.
- **Best Time to Plant Outdoors:** The ideal time to plant Holy Basil outdoors is after the last frost in spring, typically in late April or May, when the soil has warmed up.
- **Spacing Outdoor Plants:** Space plants or seeds about 12 to 18 inches apart to allow for adequate air circulation and growth.
- **Container Use and Soil:** Holy Basil thrives in well-drained soil with a neutral pH. For container planting, use a well-aerated potting mix to prevent waterlogging.
- **Sunlight and Location:** Holy Basil requires full sun, around 6 to 8 hours of direct sunlight per day. If using artificial lighting, LED grow lights can provide the full spectrum of light needed for healthy growth.
- **Watering:** Water the plants regularly to keep the soil moist but not waterlogged. Allow the top inch of soil to dry out before watering again.
- **Feeding:** Fertilize with a balanced, organic fertilizer every 4 to 6 weeks during the growing season to support growth.

- **Pruning and Maintenance:** Regularly snip off dead flowers to encourage bushier growth and prevent the plant from flowering too early, which can reduce leaf production.
- **Pest and Disease Management:** Watch for common pests like aphids and spider mites. Use organic pest control methods and ensure good air circulation to prevent fungal diseases.
- **Overwintering:** In colder climates, Holy Basil can be moved indoors or treated as an annual, as it does not tolerate frost.
- **Propagation:** Propagate by seed or cuttings in early spring to expand your Holy Basil collection.
- **Harvesting:** Leaves can be harvested throughout the growing season once the plant has become established. Use leaves fresh or dried in teas, cooking, or for medicinal purposes.
- **Climate Considerations:** Holy Basil prefers warm, tropical to subtropical climates but can be grown in temperate zones during the warmer months. It does not thrive in cold conditions, so in cooler climates, it should be grown in pots that can be brought indoors during winter.

How to Use Holy Basil

Herbal Teas or Infusions: Soak the leaves in hot water for about 5 to 10 minutes to make a soothing tea, which is commonly consumed for its stress-relieving and antioxidant properties.

Tinctures: Holy Basil leaves are soaked in alcohol to extract their active compounds, creating a concentrated tincture that can be used for its therapeutic effects.

Salves-Topical Applications: The leaves are infused into oils to make creams or ointments, applied to the skin to soothe irritations or wounds.

Compresses: Infused leaves or essential oils are used in compresses to reduce inflammation and soothe skin conditions.

Aromatherapy & Essential Oils: Holy Basil oil is used in diffusers or applied topically (diluted in a carrier oil) for its calming and antimicrobial properties.

Decoctions: A strong tea made by boiling the leaves for an extended period, often used in traditional medicine to support respiratory health.

Syrups: The extract of Holy Basil leaves is combined with sugar to make a syrup, used to soothe sore throats or coughs.

Culinary Uses: Fresh or dried leaves are used to flavor dishes, particularly in Thai and Indian cuisine, imparting a unique taste and offering health benefits.

Ease to Grow: 2-4, Low Maintenance

Holy Basil is relatively easy to grow, thriving in warm conditions with sufficient sunlight. It requires regular watering but is otherwise low maintenance, making it a good choice for both beginner and experienced gardeners.

Hops

Scientifically as Humulus Lupulus, are perennial plants famous for their use in beer production, adding flavor and preserving qualities. Originating in Europe, Asia, and North America, hops grow in temperate climates, climbing and supporting themselves on structures. They are valued for their cones, which contain lupulin glands secreting acids and essential oils that impart distinctive tastes and aromas. Beyond brewing, hops have sedative and antibacterial properties, making them a subject of interest in herbal medicine.

Nervous System
Sleep and anxiety: Hops act as a natural sedative, helping to improve sleep quality and reduce anxiety levels.

Digestive System
Stomach: They aid in digestion by stimulating gastric juice production and reducing spasms in the digestive tract.

Reproductive System
Hormonal balance: Hops contain phytoestrogens that can help in regulating menstrual cycles and reducing menopausal symptoms.

Cardiovascular System
Blood vessels: The anti-inflammatory properties of hops contribute to cardiovascular health by helping to prevent the hardening of arteries.

How to Grow Hops

- **Selecting the Right Variety:** For brewing, Cascade and Centennial are popular hop varieties. For ornamental purposes, Golden Hops offer visual appeal. Starting from rhizomes (root cuttings) is common, but seeds can be used for breeding purposes. Purchase rhizomes or seeds from reputable nurseries or online stores specializing in hop plants.

- **Best Time to Plant Outdoors:** Plant hops in early spring, after the last frost, when the soil is workable. This gives the plant a full growing season to establish.
- **Spacing Outdoor Plants:** Plant hop rhizomes (horizontal underground stems) about 3 to 5 feet apart in rows, with 7 to 8 feet between the rows to allow for growth and air circulation.
- **Container Use and Soil:** Hops can grow in large containers but thrive in well-drained, loamy soil with a pH between 6.0 and 7.5. Ensure the container is large enough to accommodate the root system and provide adequate drainage.
- **Sunlight and Location:** Hops need full sun, requiring at least 6-8 hours of direct sunlight daily. If using artificial lighting, full-spectrum LED grow lights are effective, mimicking natural sunlight.
- **Watering:** Keep the soil consistently moist but not waterlogged. Hops require more water during the growing and flowering stages.
- **Feeding:** Apply a balanced fertilizer in early spring and again in early summer to support growth and hop cone development.
- **Pruning and Maintenance:** In the first year, allow plants to grow without pruning to strengthen the root system. In subsequent years, trim in early spring to select 3-5 strong bines (growing vines) per plant. Snip off dead flowers to encourage growth.
- **Pest and Disease Management:** Watch for aphids, spider mites, and powdery mildew. Use organic pesticides or introduce beneficial insects. Remove and destroy infected plant parts to control disease spread.
- **Overwintering:** In colder climates, cover the base of the plant with mulch to protect the roots from freezing temperatures.

- **Propagation:** Propagate by dividing rhizomes in the dormant season (late winter to early spring).
- **Harvesting:** Harvest hops when they are dry and papery, usually in late summer. The cones should be fragrant and spring back when squeezed. Use fresh or dry them for later use.
- **Climate Considerations:** Hops grow best in climates with cold winters and long summer days. They need a dormant period with chilling to thrive, avoiding extremely hot or tropical climates.

How to Use Hops

Herbal Teas or Infusions: Soak hops in hot water to make a calming tea. The bitter taste can be mellowed with honey or blended with other herbs.

Tinctures: Soak hops in alcohol to extract their calming and sleep-inducing properties, creating a potent tincture for medicinal use.

Salves-Topical Applications: Hops can be infused into oils to make creams or ointments, offering anti-inflammatory benefits for skin irritations and aches.

Compresses: A cloth soaked in a strong hops infusion can be applied to the skin to soothe inflammation and relieve pain.

Herbal Baths: Adding hops to bathwater can create a relaxing soak, aiding in stress relief and skin health.

Steam Inhalation: Inhaling steam from a decoction of hops can help clear nasal passages and relax the mind.

Decoctions: Boiling hops in water makes a strong decoction that can be used for therapeutic baths or as a base for syrups.

Syrups: Concentrated hops decoction sweetened with sugar or honey creates a syrup to ease coughs and sore throats.

Gargles & Mouthwashes: A cooled hops infusion can be used as a gargle or mouthwash to soothe throat irritation and improve oral health.

Powders: Dried and powdered hops can be used in capsule form for dietary supplements or as a seasoning in culinary preparations.

Juices: Fresh hops are rarely juiced due to their intense bitterness but may be used in small quantities in herbal juice blends.

Culinary Uses: Hops are primarily used in brewing beer for flavoring, but young hop shoots can be cooked and eaten like asparagus.

Ease to Grow: 3-6, Medium Maintenance

Hops are relatively easy to grow, thriving in well-drained soil and full sun. They require support for climbing and benefit from regular watering and pruning to encourage healthy growth and optimal cone production.

Horehound

(Marrubium vulgare) is a perennial herb from the mint family, known for its bitter taste and medicinal properties. It thrives in dry, sandy soils and has been used traditionally in Europe and the Americas. The plant features wooly leaves and white flowers, and its extracts are commonly found in cough syrups and lozenges. Horehound is reputed for its effectiveness in treating respiratory and digestive ailments, due to its expectorant, stimulant, and anti-inflammatory properties.

Respiratory System

Lungs: Horehound acts as an expectorant, aiding in the clearance of mucus and easing coughs, supporting lung health.

Airways: Helps soothe irritated respiratory tracts, reducing the severity and frequency of coughing episodes.

Digestive System

Stomach: The herb stimulates appetite and aids in digestion by promoting the secretion of digestive juices.

Intestines: It can relieve intestinal gas and discomfort, improving overall digestive function.

Immune System

General Immunity: Horehound may bolster the immune system by enhancing the body's defense mechanisms against common infections and pathogens. Its antimicrobial properties help in fighting off bacteria and viruses, contributing to overall health and disease prevention.

How to Grow Horehound

- **Selecting the Right Variety:** Horehound typically has only one commonly grown variety, Marrubium Vulgare. It's best started from seeds or cuttings. Seeds can be purchased from online garden centers or local nurseries. For medicinal purposes, ensure you get the true horehound variety.
- **Best Time to Plant Outdoors:** Plant horehound seeds or starts in early spring after the last frost. The plant tolerates cold well, but young plants should be established before winter.

- **Spacing Outdoor Plants:** Space plants or seeds about 18 to 24 inches apart to allow for their growth into bushy spreads.

- **Container Use and Soil:** Horehound thrives in well-drained soil with a neutral to alkaline pH. In containers, use a standard potting mix with added perlite for better drainage.

- **Sunlight and Location:** Requires full sun, meaning at least six hours of direct sunlight daily. Can tolerate partial shade but may not flower as prolifically. In regions with intense sun, light afternoon shade is beneficial.

- **Watering:** Water young plants regularly until established. Mature Horehound is drought-tolerant and needs only occasional watering during extremely dry periods.

- **Feeding:** Horehound generally does not require frequent fertilization. A light application of a balanced fertilizer in the spring can support growth.

- **Pruning and Maintenance:** Snip off dead flowers to promote bushier growth and prevent the plant from flowering too early. Regular trimming helps maintain shape.

- **Pest and Disease Management:** Horehound is not commonly affected by pests or diseases. However, watch for common garden pests and treat with appropriate organic methods if necessary.

- **Overwintering:** In colder climates, horehound will die back to the ground and return in spring. No special winter care is needed.

- **Propagation:** Propagate by seed in the spring or by division in spring or fall. Cuttings can also be taken in late spring or early summer.

- **Harvesting:** Harvest leaves and flowering tops as the plant begins to bloom, usually in late spring to early summer. These parts are used for medicinal purposes. Dry them for later use or use fresh.

- **Climate Considerations:** Thrives in temperate climates but can adapt to various conditions. Avoid waterlogged areas and extremely hot, humid environments. Prefers a climate where it can receive full sun most of the day.

How to Use Horehound

Herbal Teas or Infusions: Horehound leaves are soaked in hot water to make a bitter tea, often sweetened with honey, used for its expectorant properties.

Tinctures: The leaves and flowers are soaked in alcohol to extract the active ingredients, creating a tincture that can help with digestive and respiratory issues.

Salves-Topical Applications: Crushed leaves are mixed into a base of wax and oils to make salves or ointments applied to the skin for irritation and inflammation.

Decoctions: The leaves are boiled in water for a long time to make a strong decoction, used to relieve respiratory ailments.

Syrups: The extract of horehound is mixed with sugar or honey to make a syrup that soothes sore throats and coughs.

Gargles & Mouthwashes: A cooled tea or decoction can be used as a gargle or mouthwash to treat sore throats and mouth ulcers.

Powders: Dried horehound leaves are ground into a powder, which can be used to make capsules or mixed with water to create a paste for topical use.

Ease to Grow: 2-3, Low Maintenance

Horehound is a hardy perennial herb that's easy to grow, requiring minimal care once established. It thrives in well-drained soil and full sun but can tolerate poor soil and drought conditions. Regular harvesting encourages new growth and prevents the plant from becoming woody (stunted growth).

Horsetail

Also known by its scientific name Equisetum Arvense, is an ancient herb that actually predates the dinosaurs! Characterized by its reed-like stems and that it lacks true leaves or flowers. Horsetail is rich in silica, minerals, and antioxidants, making it beneficial for several physiological systems. It is particularly noted for its ability to improve the health of the urinary tract, skin, hair, nails, and bones due to its nutrient content.

Digestive System

Stomach: Horsetail can aid in soothing gastrointestinal discomfort and reducing inflammation in the digestive tract.

Urinary System

Kidneys: It acts as a diuretic, increasing urine flow to help flush out kidney stones and urinary tract infections.

Bladder: Horsetail may soothe bladder irritation and help in the treatment of incontinence and bladder weakness.

Skin and Integumentary System

Skin: The silica in horsetail helps improve skin elasticity and the healing of wounds, cuts, and burns.

Hair: Its nutrients strengthen hair follicles, promoting hair growth and improving hair health.

Respiratory System

Lungs: Horsetail has been used to treat respiratory issues, acting as an expectorant to clear excess mucus and relieve congestion.

Skeletal System

Bones: Horsetail's high silica content contributes to bone density, promoting bone growth and repair, and may help prevent osteoporosis.

How to Grow Horsetail

- **Selecting the Right Variety:** Horsetail (Equisetum Arvense) is the common variety used for medicinal purposes. It's preferable to propagate horsetail through division or spores rather than seeds, as it doesn't produce conventional seeds. You can purchase horsetail plants or spores from specialty herb nurseries or online stores specializing in medicinal plants.
- **Best Time to Plant Outdoors:** Plant horsetail in the spring or autumn when the weather is cooler, as it prefers mild temperatures for initial growth.
- **Spacing Outdoor Plants:** Space horsetail plants or clusters about 1 to 2 feet apart to allow room for spread, as they can grow aggressively.
- **Container Use and Soil:** Horsetail thrives in moist, well-draining soil with a slightly acidic to neutral pH. When grown in containers, use a mix of peat, sand, and garden soil to ensure adequate drainage and mimic its natural habitat.
- **Sunlight and Location:** Horsetail prefers partial shade but can tolerate full sun if kept moist. It requires at least 4 to 6

hours of sunlight daily. If using artificial lighting, fluorescent grow lights are suitable.

- **Watering:** Maintain consistent moisture, especially during dry periods, as horsetail thrives in wet environments.
- **Feeding:** Horsetail requires little to no fertilization. If necessary, a light application of a balanced, slow-release fertilizer in the spring can promote growth.
- **Pruning and Maintenance:** Regularly check for and remove any yellowed stems. Snip off any dead stems to encourage healthy new growth.
- **Pest and Disease Management:** Horsetail is generally pest-resistant but watch for rust and fungal diseases. Remove affected parts and improve air circulation to manage these issues.
- **Overwintering:** Horsetail is hardy and typically survives winter without special care. In extremely cold areas, mulching can help protect the roots.
- **Propagation:** Propagate by dividing the rhizomes (underground stems) in spring or autumn. Plant them immediately in moist soil.
- **Harvesting:** Harvest the aerial parts of horsetail in summer when the stems are green and vibrant. Use them fresh or dry them for later use. Horsetail is valued for its minerals, especially silica, which is beneficial for bone and skin health.
- **Climate Considerations:** Horsetail adapts well to a variety of climates but thrives best in temperate regions where it can grow in wet, marshy conditions. Avoid extremely hot, dry environments.

How to Use Horsetail

Herbal Teas or Infusions: Horsetail is often soaked in hot water to create a tea or infusion, believed to support urinary tract health and provide minerals like silica.

Decoctions: A stronger preparation than tea, horsetail is boiled to extract its beneficial compounds, used to support nail, hair, and bone health.

Powders: Dried and ground horsetail is made into a powder, which can be added to smoothies or capsules for supplemental intake.

Ease to Grow: 2-4, Low Maintenance

Horsetail is a robust plant that thrives in wet, sandy soil and spreads quickly. Its ease of growth and low maintenance make it a persistent garden inhabitant, often growing in large patches.

Hyssop

A herbaceous plant known for its aromatic leaves and vibrant flowers, often used in culinary and medicinal applications. Traditionally, hyssop has been associated with purification and is mentioned in ancient texts for its cleansing properties. It thrives in well-drained soil with full sun exposure and is recognized for its minty, somewhat bitter flavor. Hyssop's essential oils are extracted for various uses, including aromatherapy and natural remedies.

Respiratory System

Lungs: Hyssop's expectorant properties help clear mucus, making it beneficial for alleviating coughs and easing congestion in the respiratory tract.

Digestive System

Stomach: It aids digestion, reduces gas, and soothes abdominal discomfort, promoting overall digestive health.

Cardiovascular System

Blood Circulation: Hyssop can improve circulation, contributing to better heart health and reducing hypertension.

Immune System

Immune Response: The antiviral and antimicrobial effects of hyssop boost the immune system, helping to fight off infections.

Skin and Integumentary System

Skin: Its antiseptic and healing properties make hyssop useful in treating skin irritations, wounds, and infections.

How to Grow Hyssop

- **Selecting the Right Variety:** Hyssop has a few varieties like 'Blue Flower' and 'Pink Flower'. Seeds are commonly used to start plants, available in nurseries or online. Decide based on the color and plant size you prefer for your garden.

- **Best Time to Plant Outdoors:** Plant hyssop seeds or starts in the spring after the last frost to give them a full growing season to establish.
- **Spacing Outdoor Plants:** Space plants or seeds about 12 to 18 inches apart to ensure adequate airflow and reduce competition for nutrients.
- **Container Use and Soil:** Hyssop grows well in containers using well-draining soil. A standard potting mix is suitable for pots and outdoor planting.
- **Sunlight and Location:** Requires full sun, meaning at least 6 to 8 hours of direct sunlight daily. If using artificial light, LED grow lights can mimic natural sunlight.
- **Watering:** Water regularly to keep the soil moist but not waterlogged. Reduce watering frequency once the plant is established.
- **Feeding:** Apply a balanced liquid fertilizer monthly during the growing season to support healthy growth.
- **Pruning and Maintenance:** Snip off dead flowers to encourage new growth and prevent the plant from flowering too early.
- **Pest and Disease Management:** Watch for aphids and treat with neem oil or insecticidal soap. Practice crop rotation to prevent soil-borne diseases.
- **Overwintering:** In colder climates, mulch around the base to protect roots from freezing temperatures.
- **Propagation:** Propagate hyssop by seed, division, or cuttings in late spring or early summer to allow time for root development before winter.
- **Harvesting:** Leaves and flowers can be harvested just before the plant blooms for the most potent flavor and medicinal properties. Use shears to cut stems cleanly.

- **Climate Considerations:** Thrives in temperate climates with cold winters and warm summers. Avoid overly wet or humid conditions to prevent root rot and other moisture-related diseases.

How to Use Hyssop

Herbal Teas or Infusions: Hyssop leaves are soaked in hot water to create an aromatic tea, known for its soothing and digestive benefits.

Tinctures: The leaves and flowers are soaked in alcohol to extract their active compounds, used for respiratory and digestive support.

Salves-Topical Applications: Hyssop infused oil is used in salves for its antiseptic and anti-inflammatory properties to heal skin irritations and wounds.

Decoctions: The plant is simmered in water for a long time to extract deeper flavors and medicinal properties, often used for coughs and sore throats.

Syrups: Hyssop is boiled with sugar or honey to create a syrup, helping soothe sore throats and coughs.

Culinary Uses: Fresh or dried hyssop leaves are used as a herb in cooking, adding a bitter, minty flavor to dishes like soups and salads.

Ease to Grow: 2-4, Low Maintenance

Hyssop is a hardy perennial herb that is relatively easy to grow, requiring minimal care. It thrives in well-drained soil and full sun, and once established, it is drought-tolerant and low maintenance, making it suitable for novice gardeners.

Lady's Mantle

Scientifically known as Alchemilla vulgaris, is a perennial herb cherished for its unique, fan-shaped, and dew-catching leaves. This plant has a rich history in herbal medicine, dating back to medieval times when it was used for various ailments. It grows in a rosette form, producing greenish-yellow flowers. Lady's Mantle prefers cool climates and thrives in well-drained soil, partial shade to full sun. It's known for its astringent (restrict or tighten tissue) properties due to the tannins present, making it beneficial for treating wounds and gastrointestinal issues.

Reproductive System

Uterus: It is traditionally used to regulate menstrual cycles, reduce menstrual pain, and aid in the recovery postpartum.

Digestive System

Stomach: Lady's Mantle's astringent properties help to reduce gastrointestinal discomfort, alleviate diarrhea, and soothe inflammation.

Skin and Integumentary System

Skin: The herb's astringent and healing properties make it beneficial for treating cuts, wounds, and skin irritations, promoting faster healing and reducing inflammation.

How to Grow Lady's Mantle

- **Selecting the Right Variety:** Lady's Mantle (Alchemilla Vulgaris) is commonly cultivated. Varieties like 'Thriller' have larger leaves and more pronounced flowers. Seeds or starts are both suitable for propagation. Check local nurseries or online stores for availability.
- **Best Time to Plant Outdoors:** Plant in early spring or fall when the weather is cool. This timing helps the plant establish without the stress of extreme heat.
- **Spacing Outdoor Plants:** Space plants about 12 to 18 inches apart to allow room for growth and air circulation, reducing the risk of disease.
- **Container Use and Soil:** Prefers well-draining soil rich in organic matter. In containers, use a loamy potting mix to ensure proper drainage and root development.
- **Sunlight and Location:** Thrives in partial shade but can tolerate full sun in cooler climates. In hotter areas, provide some afternoon shade. For artificial lighting, use grow lights that mimic natural sunlight for about 6-8 hours per day.
- **Watering:** Water regularly to keep the soil moist but not waterlogged. Reduce watering during the winter dormant period.
- **Feeding:** Apply a balanced, slow-release fertilizer in the spring to support growth and flowering.
- **Pruning and Maintenance:** Snip off dead flowers to encourage more blooms and prevent self-seeding. Trim back in late fall to tidy the plant and promote healthy spring growth.

- **Pest and Disease Management:** Monitor for common garden pests like aphids. Manage diseases like powdery mildew by ensuring good air circulation and proper watering practices.
- **Overwintering:** Lady's Mantle is hardy and generally survives winter well. In very cold climates, mulch around the base to protect roots.
- **Propagation:** Can be propagated by seed, division in spring or autumn, or by root cuttings.
- **Harvesting:** Leaves and flowers can be harvested in summer when in full bloom. They are used in herbal remedies and teas, valued for their astringent properties.
- **Climate Considerations:** Prefers temperate climates with cool summers. Not suited to hot, dry climates, unless provided with adequate shade and moisture.

How to Use Lady's Mantle

Herbal Teas or Infusions: Lady's Mantle leaves are soaked in boiling water to create a herbal tea, known for its gentle astringent properties and support for menstrual and digestive health.

Tinctures: The aerial parts of the plant are used to make a tincture, which is taken in small doses to help with digestive issues and menstrual cramps.

Salves-Topical Applications: The leaves are infused into oils to create salves and creams for treating skin irritations and wounds due to its astringent and healing properties.

Decoctions: A strong decoction can be made from the leaves, used for gargling to relieve sore throats and for topical application on skin irritations.

Gargles & Mouthwashes: The decoction is also used as a gargle or mouthwash to treat oral inflammations and sore throats.

Lady's Mantle is a hardy perennial that thrives in cool, temperate climates. It prefers partial shade and well-drained soil but can tolerate a range of conditions. Its resilience and low maintenance requirements make it a favored plant in many gardens, offering both medicinal and ornamental value.

Lavender

A very popular herb known for its fragrant purple flowers, is widely appreciated for its calming aroma and therapeutic properties. It thrives in sunny, well-drained environments and has been used for centuries in various forms such as essential oils, dried flowers, and teas. Lavender's benefits span across several physiological systems, particularly the nervous, digestive, and skin systems.

Nervous System

Brain: Lavender oil has a calming effect, reducing anxiety and improving sleep quality by inducing relaxation.

Digestive System

Stomach: It can alleviate gastrointestinal issues like bloating and indigestion by relaxing the stomach muscles and reducing inflammation.

Skin and Integumentary System

Skin: Lavender promotes wound healing, reduces inflammation, and has antiseptic properties that can treat minor burns and insect bites.

How to Grow Lavender

- **Selecting the Right Variety:** Popular varieties of Lavender include Lavandula Angustifolia (English Lavender) and Lavandula x intermedia (Lavandin). Starting from seeds can be challenging; purchasing young plants from a reputable nursery is recommended. Look for plants adapted to your climate and soil conditions.
- **Best Time to Plant Outdoors:** Plant lavender in the spring or early fall when the weather is mild. This timing allows the plant to establish itself before extreme temperatures of winter or summer.
- **Spacing Outdoor Plants:** Space plants about 18 to 24 inches apart to ensure good air circulation and prevent fungal diseases.
- **Container Use and Soil:** Lavender thrives in well-draining soil with a pH between 6.5 and 7.5. In containers, use a mix of potting soil, sand, and compost to improve drainage.
- **Sunlight and Location:** Lavender requires full sun, meaning at least 6 hours of direct sunlight daily. If using artificial lighting, LED grow lights are effective; provide 14-16 hours of light per day.
- **Watering:** Water young plants regularly until they are established. Mature lavender plants are drought-tolerant and only need watering during extended dry periods.

- **Feeding:** Lavender generally does not require frequent fertilization. Apply a light dressing of compost or slow-release fertilizer in the spring.
- **Pruning and Maintenance:** Snip off dead flowers to encourage new growth and maintain plant shape. Prune annually in the spring or fall, removing old woody stems to promote fresh growth.
- **Pest and Disease Management:** Monitor for common pests like aphids and diseases like root rot. Good air circulation and well-draining soil help prevent most issues. Treat infections early with appropriate organic or chemical treatments.
- **Overwintering:** In colder climates, protect lavender with mulch or coverings during winter to prevent frost damage.
- **Propagation:** Propagate lavender from cuttings in the late spring to early summer. Choose healthy, non-flowering stems for best results.
- **Harvesting:** Harvest lavender flowers when they are fully colored but not fully open, typically in the morning after the dew has evaporated. Flowers, leaves, and stems can be used for their scent and oils.
- **Climate Considerations:** Lavender grows best in warm, sunny climates with well-drained soil. It can tolerate some cold but prefers regions where winter temperatures do not plummet deeply and consistently.

How to Use Lavender

Herbal Teas or Infusions: Soak dried lavender flowers in hot water to create a calming tea that helps relaxation and sleep.
Tinctures: Lavender can be soaked in alcohol to create a tincture, used for its antiseptic and calming properties.

Salves-Topical Applications: Lavender oil is incorporated into creams, ointments, and poultices to soothe skin irritations, burns, and wounds.

Compresses: Soak a cloth in a lavender infusion or dilute lavender essential oil for a compress to relieve headaches or skin discomfort.

Aromatherapy & Essential Oils: Lavender oil is used in diffusers for breathing or applied directly to the skin for its relaxing and antibacterial effects.

Herbal Baths: Adding lavender flowers or oil to bathwater can promote relaxation and skin health.

Steam Inhalation: Inhaling steam infused with lavender oil can help clear nasal passages and relieve respiratory issues.

Decoctions: A strong lavender decoction can be made and used for its antiseptic and anti-inflammatory properties.

Syrups: Lavender syrup, often made from the flowers, is used to flavor food and drinks and has soothing properties.

Gargles & Mouthwashes: A lavender infusion can be used as a gargle or mouthwash to freshen breath and reduce oral bacteria.

Powders: Dried lavender can be powdered and used in cosmetics, sachets, and as a natural deodorant.

Culinary Uses: Lavender is used in culinary dishes for its unique flavor, especially in desserts and teas.

Ease to Grow: 2-4, Low Maintenance

Lavender is quite adaptable and grows well in many conditions, requiring minimal water once established and preferring full sunlight. It is resistant to most pests and diseases, making it a low-maintenance choice for both novice and experienced gardeners.

Lemon Balm

(Melissa Officinalis) is a perennial herb in the mint family, known for its lemon-scented leaves. It has been used historically in herbal medicine to improve mood, reduce stress, and aid digestion. Grows in clumps and produces small, white flowers in summer, attracting bees and other pollinators.

Digestive System

Stomach and Intestines: Lemon Balm soothes the digestive tract, reducing bloating, gas, and discomfort associated with indigestion.

Nervous System

Brain and Nerves: Acts as a mild sedative, reducing anxiety and promoting relaxation, improving sleep quality.

Respiratory System

Lungs: Lemon Balm acts as an antispasmodic (helps relieve or prevent muscle spasms or cramps), helping to soothe respiratory conditions like coughs and may alleviate symptoms of colds by reducing mucus production.

Skin and Integumentary System

Skin: Its antiviral properties make it useful for treating cold sores and other skin irritations.

Immune System

General Immunity: Its antiviral properties strengthen the body's defense against viral infections, particularly in the case of the herpes simplex virus.

How to Grow Lemon Balm

- **Selecting the Right Variety:** Lemon Balm is generally available in one common variety, Melissa Officinalis. It's preferable to start with seeds or starts, both methods are effective. Seeds and plants can be purchased from nurseries, garden centers, or online stores.
- **Best Time to Plant Outdoors:** The ideal time to plant Lemon Balm outdoors is in the spring after the last frost. This gives ample time to establish before winter.
- **Spacing Outdoor Plants:** Space Lemon Balm plants or seeds about 18 to 24 inches apart to allow for full growth and adequate air circulation.
- **Container Use and Soil:** Lemon Balm thrives in containers with well-draining soil. For potting, use a mix rich in organic matter. It prefers a slightly moist, fertile soil with a good drainage system.
- **Sunlight and Location:** Requires at least 5 hours of direct sunlight daily, and can tolerate partial shade. For artificial lighting, use grow lights positioned a few inches above the plants.

- **Watering:** Keep the soil consistently moist but not waterlogged. Water when the top inch of soil feels dry to the touch.
- **Feeding:** Apply a balanced, slow-release fertilizer at the beginning of the growing season to support growth.
- **Pruning and Maintenance:** Regularly snip off dead flowers to promote new growth and prevent the plant from flowering too early.
- **Pest and Disease Management:** Monitor for aphids and spider mites. Use neem oil or insecticidal soap to manage infestations. Look out for powdery mildew and treat with fungicidal sprays if necessary.
- **Overwintering:** In colder climates, mulch around the base to protect roots in winter. Potted plants should be moved indoors before the first frost.
- **Propagation:** Propagate by seed, division, or stem cuttings in the spring or early summer.
- **Harvesting:** Leaves can be harvested at any time. For the best flavor, harvest in the morning after dew has evaporated. Leaves and stems are used for their medicinal and culinary properties.
- **Climate Considerations:** Lemon Balm prefers a temperate climate. It grows best in areas with cool summers and mild winters. Avoid extremely hot, dry conditions.

How to Use Lemon Balm

Herbal Teas or Infusions: Lemon Balm leaves are soaked in boiling water for about 5 to 10 minutes to create a calming tea that aids digestion and relieves stress.

Tinctures: The leaves are soaked in alcohol to extract the active compounds, creating a concentrated liquid used for its sedative and digestive properties.

Salves-Topical Applications: Crushed leaves are mixed into creams or ointments for treating cold sores, insect bites, and minor wounds due to its antiviral and antibacterial nature.

Compresses: A cloth soaked in lemon balm tea can be applied to areas of the skin for relief from pain, swelling, or to aid in healing.

Decoctions: Boiling the plant in water makes a strong liquid extract used for treating colds and flu, due to its antiviral effects.

Syrups: The extract is mixed with sugar or honey to create a syrup that soothes sore throats and coughs.

Gargles & Mouthwashes: A tea made from the leaves is used to gargle for relieving sore throats and mouth ulcers due to its soothing properties.

Culinary Uses: Fresh or dried lemon balm leaves are used in cooking for flavoring dishes and drinks with a mild, lemony taste.

Ease to Grow: 2-3, Low Maintenance

Lemon Balm is a hardy perennial herb that thrives in partial shade to full sun and well-draining soil, making it a low-maintenance choice for both novice and experienced gardeners. Its resilience and ease of care make it a popular plant in many gardens.

Lemon Verbena

Scientifically known as Aloysia Citrodora, a fragrant perennial shrub native to South America, known for its lemon-scented leaves. It is widely cultivated for its aromatic leaves, which are used in cooking and herbal medicine. This plant grows well in warm climates and prefers full sun and well-drained soil. Lemon Verbena is not only appreciated for its delightful scent and flavor but also for its therapeutic properties. It has been used traditionally to aid digestion, reduce inflammation, and relieve stress. The leaves are often used to make teas, extracts, and essential oils.

Digestive System

Stomach: Lemon Verbena is known to alleviate indigestion and reduce gas by calming the stomach and improving digestive function.

Nervous System

Brain: The calming properties of Lemon Verbena can help reduce anxiety and stress, promoting a sense of well-being and relaxation.

Immune System

General Immunity: Lemon Verbena contains antioxidants that support the immune system by fighting free radicals and reducing inflammation.

Skin and Integumentary System

Skin: Its anti-inflammatory properties help soothe irritated skin and improve its appearance by promoting healing and reducing inflammation.

How to Grow Lemon Verbena

- **Selecting the Right Variety:** Lemon Verbena (Aloysia Citrodora) is the most common variety with its lemon-scented leaves. It is usually propagated from cuttings rather than seeds to maintain desirable traits. Starts or young plants are preferable for a quicker establishment. Available at nurseries or online garden centers.
- **Best Time to Plant Outdoors:** Plant in late spring or early summer, once the risk of frost has passed, to allow the plant to establish before colder weather.
- **Spacing Outdoor Plants:** Space plants about 18 to 24 inches apart to ensure adequate airflow and sunlight penetration.
- **Container Use and Soil:** Prefers well-draining soil with a neutral to slightly alkaline pH. Suitable for container gardening, ensure pots have drainage holes and use a light, loamy potting mix.
- **Sunlight and Location:** Requires full sun, about 6 to 8 hours of direct sunlight daily. Can tolerate partial shade. In regions with intense heat, some afternoon shade can prevent scorching.
- **Watering:** Water regularly but allow the soil to dry out between watering to prevent root rot. Less water is needed in the winter months.
- **Feeding:** Apply a balanced, slow-release fertilizer in early spring to support growth. Monthly liquid feed during the growing season can promote lush foliage.

- **Pruning and Maintenance:** Snip off dead flowers to encourage new growth and maintain plant shape. Prune heavily in early spring to promote vigorous growth.
- **Pest and Disease Management:** Watch for aphids and spider mites. Use insecticidal soap or neem oil for treatment. Root rot can occur in overly moist soil, ensure good drainage.
- **Overwintering:** In colder climates, bring indoors or provide mulch for root protection. Prefers a cool, frost-free area during winter.
- **Propagation:** Propagate by stem cuttings in late spring or early summer. Cut a 6-inch stem, remove the bottom leaves, and plant in well-draining soil.
- **Harvesting:** Leaves can be harvested anytime during the growing season. However, they're most aromatic just before the plant flowers. Use leaves fresh or dried for teas and culinary uses.
- **Climate Considerations:** Thrives in warm, temperate climates. Performs best in areas with clear, distinct seasons and relatively low humidity. Does not tolerate extreme cold well.

How to Use Lemon Verbena

Herbal Teas or Infusions: Lemon Verbena leaves are soaked in hot water for several minutes to make a fragrant herbal tea that can aid digestion and promote relaxation.

Tinctures: Fresh or dried leaves are soaked in alcohol to extract the plant's beneficial compounds, creating a concentrated liquid used for its therapeutic properties.

Salves-Topical Applications: The leaves are infused in oil to make salves or ointments for skin irritations and to promote wound healing.

Compresses: A cloth soaked in a decoction of the plant is applied to the skin to reduce inflammation and soothe skin conditions.

Aromatherapy & Essential Oils: Lemon Verbena's essential oil is used in aromatherapy for its calming and uplifting effects, inhaled directly or applied topically when diluted.

Herbal Baths: Leaves are added to bathwater or used in a bath sachet to soothe and relax the body and mind.

Steam Inhalation: Inhaling the steam from a hot water infusion of the leaves can relieve nasal congestion and respiratory issues.

Decoctions: The leaves are boiled in water for a period to extract deeper flavors and benefits, used for digestive ailments.

Syrups: The plant's extract is mixed with sugar or honey to create a syrup that can soothe sore throats and coughs.

Culinary Uses: Fresh or dried Lemon Verbena leaves are used to flavor dishes, teas, and desserts with their citrusy aroma and taste.

Ease to Grow: 3-5, Low Maintenance

Lemon Verbena is fairly easy to grow, requiring full sun, well-drained soil, and regular watering. It thrives in warm climates but can be grown in containers in colder regions so move indoors during winter.

Lemongrass

A perennial grass native to tropical regions, and widely cultivated for its aromatic stalks used in cooking and herbal medicine. Known for its citrus scent, it is a staple in Asian cuisine and is also valued for its therapeutic properties. Lemongrass contains essential oils, including citral, which have been found to have anti-inflammatory, antibacterial, and antifungal effects.

Digestive System

Stomach: Lemongrass promotes healthy digestion by relieving bloating, cramps, and indigestion, and stimulates bowel function.

Nervous System

Brain: It has a calming effect, reducing stress and anxiety, improving mood, and aiding in better sleep quality.

Skin and Integumentary System

Skin: Its antimicrobial and anti-inflammatory properties help in treating skin infections and improving overall skin health.

Respiratory System

Airways: Lemongrass acts as an expectorant, helping to clear mucus and relieve respiratory conditions like colds and flu.

How to Grow Lemongrass

- **Selecting the Right Variety:** Common varieties of Lemongrass include Cymbopogon Citratus and Cymbopogon Flexuosus. It's typically grown from stalks rather than seeds, which can be purchased at nurseries or online garden shops.
- **Best Time to Plant Outdoors:** Plant lemongrass in spring, after the last frost, when the soil has warmed up.
- **Spacing Outdoor Plants:** Space plants or stalks about 24 inches apart to give each plant room to grow.

- **Container Use and Soil:** Lemongrass thrives in large pots with well-draining soil; it prefers loamy or sandy soil rich in organic matter.
- **Sunlight and Location:** Requires full sun, at least 6 hours of direct sunlight daily. Can be grown under artificial grow lights if natural light is insufficient.
- **Watering:** Water regularly to keep the soil moist but not waterlogged. Lemongrass prefers consistent moisture.
- **Feeding:** Fertilize with a balanced, slow-release fertilizer every few months to support growth.
- **Pruning and Maintenance:** Snip off dead leaves and stalks to encourage new growth. Lemongrass doesn't typically flower in most climates, so deadheading isn't a concern (snipping off of dead flowers).
- **Pest and Disease Management:** Watch for signs of rust or fungal diseases. Treat with appropriate fungicides and keep the area around plants clean to prevent issues.
- **Overwintering:** In cooler climates, move pots indoors or protect outdoor plants with mulch to overwinter.
- **Propagation:** Propagate by dividing the root ball or planting fresh stalks that have visible growth nodes.
- **Harvesting:** Harvest lemongrass stalks by cutting them close to the ground level. Leaves and stalks are used in cooking for their flavor.
- **Climate Considerations:** Thrives in warm, humid environments but can be grown in cooler areas with winter protection or as an annual. Avoid cold, frost-prone regions for outdoor planting.

How to Use Lemongrass

Herbal Teas or Infusions: Lemongrass leaves are soaked in boiling water to create a refreshing tea known for its digestive and calming properties.

Tinctures: The stalks of Lemongrass are macerated in alcohol to extract essential oils, used for their therapeutic benefits.

Salves-Topical Applications: Lemongrass oil is infused in creams or ointments for its antibacterial and anti-inflammatory properties, aiding in skin care and muscle relaxation.

Decoctions: Boiling Lemongrass for an extended period makes a strong decoction, used for its intense flavor in culinary dishes and therapeutic properties.

Juices: Fresh Lemongrass stalks are juiced or crushed to extract the liquid, used for its digestive and flavor-enhancing benefits.

Culinary Uses: Lemongrass is widely used in cooking for its citrus flavor, particularly in Asian cuisine, to season soups, teas, and curries.

Ease to Grow: 3-5, Low Maintenance

Lemongrass is a resilient plant that thrives in warm, sunny conditions with regular watering. It's relatively easy to grow in the right climate or indoors with sufficient light, making it a low-maintenance choice for gardeners.

Licorice

Scientifically known as Glycyrrhiza Glabra, is a perennial herb native to parts of Europe and Asia. It has a long history of use in traditional medicine and is renowned for its sweet flavor, derived from the compound "glycyrrhizin", which is many times sweeter than sugar. Licorice root is used in various forms, including teas, candies, and as a flavoring agent in foods and beverages. Medicinally, it is utilized for its anti-inflammatory, antimicrobial, and soothing properties. Often used to treat gastrointestinal issues, respiratory conditions, and skin ailments, among other health concerns.

Digestive System

Stomach lining: Licorice soothes the stomach lining, aids in healing ulcers, and reduces gastric inflammation.

Endocrine System

Adrenal glands: Licorice supports adrenal gland function, helping to sustain adequate cortisol levels and reduce stress effects.

Respiratory System

Lungs: Acts as an expectorant, helping to clear mucus and relieve symptoms of coughs and sore throats.

How to Grow Licorice

- **Selecting the Right Variety:** Licorice is typically grown from the species Glycyrrhiza Glabra. It's preferable to start with root cuttings or seeds, which can be purchased from specialized herb nurseries or online stores. Ensure you acquire a variety suited to your climate and soil conditions.

- **Best Time to Plant Outdoors:** Plant licorice in the spring or fall when temperatures are mild. This timing helps the plants to establish without the stress of extreme heat or cold.
- **Spacing Outdoor Plants:** Space plants or seeds about 3 feet apart to allow room for growth and ensure good air circulation, which is vital for healthy development.
- **Container Use and Soil:** Licorice thrives in deep, fertile, well-drained soil with a pH between 6.0 and 7.5. While it prefers open ground, large containers can be used if they provide ample space for the extensive root system.
- **Sunlight and Location:** Licorice plants need full sun to partial shade, with at least 6 hours of sunlight daily. If using artificial lighting, full-spectrum LED grow lights are effective.
- **Watering:** Keep the soil consistently moist but not waterlogged. Licorice requires regular watering, especially during dry spells, to maintain healthy growth.
- **Feeding:** Apply a balanced, slow-release fertilizer in the spring to support growth throughout the growing season.
- **Pruning and Maintenance:** Snip off dead flowers to encourage more robust growth. Regularly check for and remove any yellowed leaves or signs of disease.
- **Pest and Disease Management:** Monitor for common pests like aphids and diseases such as root rot. Use organic pest control methods and ensure good drainage to prevent disease.
- **Overwintering:** In colder regions, mulch heavily around the base of the plant to protect the roots from freezing temperatures.
- **Propagation:** Propagate licorice by dividing the roots in early spring or late fall, ensuring each division has several growth buds.

- **Harvesting:** The roots are harvested in the fall of the third or fourth year. Dig up the long roots, wash them, and dry them for use in teas, tinctures, or powders.
- **Climate Considerations:** Licorice grows best in climates with hot summers and cool winters. It needs a full growing season of warm weather to develop fully but does not fare well in extreme heat without adequate water.

How to Use Licorice

Herbal Teas or Infusions: Licorice root is commonly soaked in hot water to make a sweet, soothing tea, often used to support digestive health and soothe sore throats.

Tinctures: The roots are extracted into alcohol to create a tincture, offering a concentrated form used for various therapeutic purposes, especially for digestive and respiratory support.

Decoctions: Licorice root is boiled in water for a long time to make a decoction, intensifying its medicinal properties, particularly for treating stomach ulcers and respiratory ailments.

Syrups: Licorice is used in syrups to ease coughs and sore throats due to its expectorant and soothing properties.

Powders: Dried licorice root is ground into a powder, which can be used for its health benefits in capsules or as a food spice.

Culinary Uses: Licorice is also used to flavor foods and beverages, including candies, desserts, and teas, imparting a distinct sweet taste.

Ease to Grow: 3-6, Medium Maintenance

A hardy plant that can be somewhat challenging to grow due to its need for specific soil conditions and a long growing season. It does prefer full sun and well-drained soil. With proper care, it grows into a robust plant that can be harvested for its sweet-tasting roots.

Lovage

A perennial herb valued for its aromatic leaves, seeds, and roots. It has been used traditionally in European cuisine and herbal medicine, often likened to celery in flavor. Lovage grows tall, with deep green leaves and yellow flowers. It's not only cultivated for its taste but also for its potential health benefits, particularly in digestive and urinary systems.

Digestive System

Stomach and Intestines: Lovage may alleviate symptoms of indigestion, reduce flatulence, and stimulate appetite due to its carminative properties (ability to relieve gastrointestinal discomfort, particularly bloating, gas, and indigestion).

Urinary System

Kidneys and Bladder: Acts as a diuretic, helping to increase urine production and relieve fluid retention, potentially supporting kidney function and urinary tract health.

How to Grow Lovage

- **Selecting the Right Variety:** Lovage is typically grown from one main species, Levisticum Officinale. Start with seeds or young plants, which can be purchased from nurseries or online garden shops. Both seeds and starts are effective, but starting with young plants can give a quicker start.

- **Best Time to Plant Outdoors:** Plant Lovage in early spring after the last frost. The plant prefers cooler temperatures for germination and early growth.
- **Spacing Outdoor Plants:** Space lovage plants or seeds about 2 to 3 feet apart, as it grows tall and bushy, requiring room to expand.
- **Container Use and Soil:** Lovage can also grow in large containers. Use well-draining soil, rich in organic matter. Outdoor garden soil should also be fertile and retain moisture without becoming waterlogged.
- **Sunlight and Location:** Lovage thrives in full sun to partial shade, needing at least 6 hours of sunlight daily. If using artificial lighting, LED grow lights can provide the necessary spectrum.
- **Watering:** Keep the soil consistently moist, especially during dry periods. Does not tolerate drought well.
- **Feeding:** Fertilize with a balanced, organic fertilizer in the spring and mid-summer to support growth.
- **Pruning and Maintenance:** Snip off dead flowers to encourage more leaf growth and prevent the plant from flowering too early.
- **Pest and Disease Management:** Watch for aphids and treat with neem oil if necessary. Root rot can occur in waterlogged soil, so ensure good drainage.
- **Overwintering:** In colder climates, mulch around the base to protect roots in winter. In milder climates, lovage may remain green throughout the year.
- **Propagation:** Propagate by seed or division in spring. Dividing mature plants helps rejuvenate them and control growth.

- **Harvesting:** Leaves can be harvested anytime during the growing season. For roots and seeds, harvest in the second or third year of growth. Leaves are used fresh or dried, and roots are washed and dried for medicinal use.
- **Climate Considerations:** Thrives in temperate climates with distinct seasons. Cold winters followed by warm summers are ideal, avoiding extreme heat.

How to Use Lovage

Herbal Teas or Infusions: Lovage leaves are soaked in boiling water to make a tea that can relieve digestive issues and promote kidney health.

Tinctures: The roots and leaves are used to create a tincture, aiding in digestion and respiratory health.

Decoctions: Lovage roots are boiled in water to make a decoction that helps with urinary and digestive problems.

Culinary Uses: Leaves and seeds are used in cooking for their celery-like flavor, enhancing soups, salads, and stews.

Ease to Grow: 3-5, Low Maintenance

Growing Lovage is relatively straightforward, needing regular watering and partial to full sun. It adapts well to garden soil and reseeds itself, making it a low-maintenance choice for both novice and experienced gardeners.

Maca

(Lepidium Meyenii) is a plant native to the high Andes of Peru, known for its cruciferous root, which is a significant dietary and medicinal component. Cultivated for over 2000 years, maca is utilized for its ability to enhance stamina, energy, and sexual function. Traditionally, it has been used both as food and medicine, suggesting a variety of health benefits.

Endocrine System

Hormone Balance: Maca is reputed to support the endocrine system's regulation of hormone balance, potentially aiding in alleviating symptoms related to hormonal imbalances.

Reproductive System

Libido: Maca is often hailed for its potential to increase sexual desire and function in both men and women.

Fertility: There is evidence suggesting that maca can improve fertility, particularly in men, by increasing sperm count and motility.

How to Grow Maca

- **Selecting the Right Variety:** Maca has different varieties, like black, red, and yellow maca, each with unique benefits;

black maca is known for improving stamina and memory, red maca for balancing hormones and increasing fertility, and yellow maca for general health benefits. Starting with seeds is challenging due to long germination times, so purchasing starts from a reputable supplier is preferable.

- **Best Time to Plant Outdoors:** Plant maca during spring or early summer to ensure it matures before colder temperatures set in, as it requires a full growth cycle close to its native high-altitude conditions.
- **Spacing Outdoor Plants:** Space maca plants about 12 inches apart to provide enough room for growth and ensure optimal root development.
- **Container Use and Soil:** Use large containers with well-draining soil, rich in organic matter. Maca thrives in loamy soil with good aeration and drainage, mimicking its native mountainous habitat.
- **Sunlight and Location:** Maca needs full sun, about 6 to 7 hours per day. If grown indoors, use high-output plant grow lights to mimic natural sunlight conditions.
- **Watering:** Keep the soil consistently moist but not waterlogged. Maca requires regular watering, especially during dry periods, to maintain healthy growth without over-saturating the roots.
- **Feeding:** Apply a balanced, organic fertilizer every four weeks during the growing season to provide necessary nutrients for maca's growth and root development.
- **Pruning and Maintenance:** Snip off dead flowers to encourage more growth and prevent the plant from spending energy on seed production.
- **Pest and Disease Management:** Monitor for common pests like aphids and diseases like root rot. Healthy maca plants

are resilient, but poor drainage and overwatering can lead to fungal issues, manifesting as blackened roots or wilted leaves.

- **Overwintering:** In colder climates, mulch heavily or bring containers indoors to protect maca roots from freezing temperatures, as maca is not frost-tolerant.
- **Propagation:** Propagate maca by dividing the root crowns in the late season before replanting, ensuring each new plant has part of the root and stem.
- **Harvesting:** Harvest maca roots after 7-9 months when leaves wilt, indicating root maturity. Dig up the entire plant, as the root contains the beneficial nutrients used for dietary and medicinal purposes.
- **Climate Considerations:** Maca prefers cool climates with ample sunlight, similar to its native Andean mountain environment, where it is cool but not excessively cold year-round.

How to Use Maca

Herbal Teas or Infusions: Maca root powder can be soaked in hot water to make herbal tea. The soaking process releases the nutrients, offering a tonic that supports energy and vitality.

Tinctures: A tincture can be made from maca root to concentrate its active compounds, providing a convenient, potent dosage form.

Powders: Maca root is commonly dried and ground into a powder, which can be added to smoothies, juices, or foods for nutritional supplementation.

Culinary Uses: Maca powder is often used in cooking and baking, adding a nutty flavor to various dishes and enhancing the nutritional content of meals.

Ease to Grow: 3-5, Medium Maintenance

Maca is relatively hardy but requires specific growing conditions that mimic its native high-altitude habitat. It needs well-draining soil, full sun, and cool temperatures, making it medium maintenance to cultivate successfully outside its native environment.

Marjoram

A perennial herb in the mint family, it is valued for its aromatic leaves, used in cooking and herbal medicine. It has a sweet, citrusy, and pine flavor profile. Marjoram is rich in antioxidants, vitamins, and minerals, supporting general health and well-being. Traditionally used to aid digestion, improve sleep, and relieve symptoms of various ailments.

Digestive System

Stomach: Marjoram helps to ease digestion, reduce stomach cramps, and alleviate gas and bloating.

Nervous System

Brain: Marjoram oil can have a calming effect, reducing stress and anxiety levels, thereby improving mental well-being.

Respiratory System

Airways: Marjoram soothes the respiratory system by acting as an expectorant, effectively clearing mucus and easing cough symptoms, aiding in more comfortable breathing.

How to Grow Marjoram

- **Selecting the Right Variety:** Marjoram comes in several varieties like sweet marjoram (most common) and pot marjoram. Sweet marjoram is preferred for its flavor and aroma. It's best to start with seeds or seedlings, which can be purchased online or at a local nursery. Ensure the seeds or plants are from a reputable source to guarantee quality.
- **Best Time to Plant Outdoors:** Plant marjoram in spring after the last frost. This herb prefers warm temperatures and will thrive when planted in a season with ample growth time before winter.
- **Spacing Outdoor Plants:** Space marjoram plants or seeds about 8 to 10 inches apart to ensure they have room to spread and receive adequate air circulation.
- **Container Use and Soil:** Marjoram grows well in containers with well-draining soil. A standard potting mix amended with compost is ideal. Ensure pots have drainage holes to prevent waterlogging.
- **Sunlight and Location:** Marjoram needs at least 6 hours of sunlight daily. It prefers full sun but can tolerate partial shade. If using artificial lighting, LED grow lights are efficient, providing the necessary light spectrum.
- **Watering:** Water marjoram when the top inch of soil feels dry. Avoid overwatering, as marjoram doesn't like soggy roots.
- **Feeding:** Fertilize marjoram sparingly; too much can diminish its flavor. Use a balanced, organic fertilizer once at the start of the growing season.

- **Pruning and Maintenance:** Regularly snip off dead flowers to encourage bushier growth and prevent the plant from flowering too early, which can reduce leaf production.
- **Pest and Disease Management:** Marjoram is relatively pest-resistant but watch for common garden pests like aphids. Treat infestations with neem oil or insecticidal soap. Prevent fungal diseases by ensuring good air circulation and not overcrowding plants.
- **Overwintering:** In colder climates, bring container-grown marjoram indoors or provide mulch for outdoor plants to protect from frost.
- **Propagation:** Propagate marjoram from cuttings in late spring or early summer to multiply your plants.
- **Harvesting:** Harvest marjoram leaves as needed, preferably in the morning after dew has evaporated. You can harvest up to one-third of the plant at a time. Use leaves fresh or dried for culinary purposes.
- **Climate Considerations:** Marjoram thrives in warm, sunny climates but can tolerate mild, cooler conditions if protected from frost and extreme cold. Avoid overly humid environments to prevent disease.

How to Use Marjoram

Herbal Teas or Infusions: Soak dried or fresh marjoram leaves in boiling water for 5-10 minutes to make a calming tea that aids digestion and soothes the stomach.

Tinctures: Marjoram leaves are soaked in alcohol to extract their active compounds, creating a tincture that can be used for digestive and nervous system support.

Salves-Topical Applications: Infused marjoram oil is used in salves and ointments to relieve muscle pain, improve circulation, and provide anti-inflammatory benefits.

Compresses: A cloth soaked in marjoram-infused water can be applied to the skin to reduce inflammation and relieve muscle or joint pain.

Decoctions: Boiling marjoram in water for an extended period makes a strong decoction that can help with respiratory conditions and digestive issues.

Syrups: Marjoram leaves are often simmered with water and sugar to create a syrup that soothes coughs and sore throats.

Gargles & Mouthwashes: A marjoram infusion is also used as a gargle or mouthwash to relieve sore throats and oral inflammation.

Culinary Uses: Extensively used in cooking to flavor soups, sauces, salads, and meat dishes, enhancing taste and aiding digestion.

Ease to Grow: 2-4, Low Maintenance

Marjoram is a hearty, low-maintenance herb that thrives in well-drained soil and full sun. It's resistant to most pests and diseases, making it an excellent choice for novice gardeners. Regular harvesting encourages growth and prevents flowering, keeping the plant lush and flavorful.

Marshmallow Root

Derived from the Althaea Officinalis plant, is renowned for its soothing and healing properties, historically used to treat various ailments. Rich in mucilage, it forms a protective layer on damaged tissues, aiding in the healing process. This herb is particularly known for its effectiveness in soothing irritated mucous membranes due to its anti-inflammatory and emollient properties.

Digestive System

Stomach: Marshmallow root coats the stomach lining, alleviating inflammation and treating ulcers by forming a protective barrier against stomach acids.

Intestines: Eases digestive issues like irritable bowel syndrome (IBS) by reducing inflammation and soothing the gut lining.

Respiratory System

Lungs: Acts as an expectorant, soothing the throat, reducing cough, and aiding in the expulsion of mucus from the respiratory tract.

Urinary System

Bladder: Marshmallow root reduces inflammation and irritation in the urinary tract, easing urination and treating urinary tract infections.

Skin and Integumentary System

Skin: Topically applied, it can soothe skin irritations, burns, and wounds by forming a protective mucilaginous layer that promotes healing and reduces inflammation.

How to Grow Marshmallow Root

- **Selecting the Right Variety:** Marshmallow Root, Althaea Officinalis, is the common variety used for medicinal purposes. It is preferable to start with seeds or root cuttings. Seeds can be purchased from online herb suppliers or garden stores.
- **Best Time to Plant Outdoors:** Plant in early spring or late autumn. The cooler temperatures help the seeds to germinate and the root cuttings to establish.
- **Spacing Outdoor Plants:** Space plants or seeds about 2 feet apart to allow room for growth and air circulation.
- **Container Use and Soil:** Prefers well-drained, loamy soil with high organic matter. Can be grown in containers with a potting mix rich in organic material.
- **Sunlight and Location:** Requires full sun to partial shade, with around 4 to 6 hours of sunlight daily. In regions with intense sun, partial shade can prevent scorching.
- **Watering:** Keep the soil consistently moist but not waterlogged. Water deeply once a week, more frequently during dry spells.
- **Feeding:** Apply a balanced liquid fertilizer monthly during the growing season to support healthy growth.
- **Pruning and Maintenance:** Regularly snip off dead flowers to encourage new growth. Remove yellowed leaves to keep the plant healthy.

- **Pest and Disease Management:** Watch for rust and leaf spot. Treat with appropriate fungicides and ensure good air circulation to prevent these diseases.
- **Overwintering:** In colder climates, mulch around the base to protect the roots during winter.
- **Propagation:** Propagate by seed in spring or by dividing the roots in autumn.
- **Harvesting:** Harvest roots in late autumn of the second year or spring of the third year. Dig up the roots, wash, and dry them for medicinal use. The leaves and flowers can also be harvested and used fresh or dried.
- **Climate Considerations:** Thrives in cool climates with adequate moisture. Can tolerate frost but not prolonged freezing temperatures. Avoid extremely hot and dry climates.

How to Use Marshmallow Root

Herbal Teas or Infusions: Soak dried marshmallow root in cold water for several hours, then heat gently to release the mucilage, which soothes the throat and digestive tract.

Tinctures: Made by soaking the root in alcohol to extract its active compounds, used for digestive and respiratory support.

Salves-Topical Applications: The mucilaginous properties of marshmallow make it ideal for creams or ointments to soothe skin irritations and inflammations.

Poultices: Crushed fresh leaves or roots applied directly to the skin to reduce inflammation and promote healing.

Compresses: A cloth soaked in an infusion of marshmallow root applied to irritated or inflamed skin to provide relief.

Decoctions: Boil the dried root to make a strong liquid extract, used for its soothing effects on the digestive and respiratory systems.

Syrups: Boil the root to make a thick, sweet liquid, often used to ease coughs and sore throats.

Gargles & Mouthwashes: A cooled tea made from the root used as a mouth rinse to soothe mouth ulcers and sore throats.

Powders: Dried and ground root used in capsule form or as a loose powder to add to food or drinks for digestive health.

Ease to Grow: 3-5, Low Maintenance

Marshmallow Root is relatively easy to grow, requiring minimal care once established. It thrives in moist, fertile soil and partial shade, making it suitable for many garden settings. Regular watering and occasional feeding will ensure healthy growth, allowing for the harvesting of its beneficial roots, leaves, and flowers.

Meadowsweet

(Filipendula Ulmaria) is a perennial herb found in damp meadows across Europe and Asia. Known for its sweet, almond-scented flowers, meadowsweet has a long history of use in traditional medicine. Its components, including salicylates, tannins, and flavonoids, contribute to its anti-inflammatory, analgesic, and diuretic properties. Meadowsweet is often used to treat digestive issues, relieve pain, and reduce fever.

Digestive System

Stomach: Meadowsweet soothes the stomach lining, helps to decrease acidity, and treats gastric ulcers by promoting mucus production.

Cardiovascular System

Blood Vessels: Its anti-inflammatory properties aid in reducing inflammation in blood vessels, improving overall cardiovascular health.

Respiratory System

Lungs: Acts as an expectorant, helping to clear mucus and relieve symptoms of colds and flu.

How to Grow Meadowsweet

- **Selecting the Right Variety:** Meadowsweet (Filipendula Ulmaria) is commonly available. Start with seeds or plants from nurseries or online stores. Both methods are suitable for growing meadowsweet.
- **Best Time to Plant Outdoors:** Plant in early spring or fall when the weather is cool. This timing helps the plant establish roots without the stress of extreme heat.
- **Spacing Outdoor Plants:** Space plants or seeds about 2 feet apart to allow for growth and air circulation, reducing the risk of disease.
- **Container Use and Soil:** Meadowsweet thrives in moist, well-drained soil. In containers, use a potting mix that retains moisture but allows excess water to drain.
- **Sunlight and Location:** Prefers full sun to partial shade. About 6 hours of sunlight daily is ideal, but it can tolerate less. For artificial lighting, use grow lights that mimic natural sunlight.

- **Watering:** Keep the soil consistently moist, especially during dry periods. Meadowsweet enjoys wet conditions but not waterlogging.
- **Feeding:** Apply a balanced liquid fertilizer monthly during the growing season to support healthy growth.
- **Pruning and Maintenance:** Snip off dead flowers to encourage more blooms and prevent the plant from flowering too early.
- **Pest and Disease Management:** Watch for rust and powdery mildew. Remove affected leaves and improve air circulation to manage these issues.
- **Overwintering:** In colder climates, mulch around the base to protect roots from freezing temperatures.
- **Propagation:** Propagate by division in spring or fall. Split large clumps into smaller sections and replant.
- **Harvesting:** Harvest leaves and flowers in summer when the plant is in bloom. These parts are used for their medicinal properties.
- **Climate Considerations:** Thrives in cool, temperate climates. Prefers areas with seasonal changes and adequate rainfall.

How to Use Meadowsweet

Herbal Teas or Infusions: Soak dried meadowsweet flowers in hot water to make a tea that can help alleviate fever and inflammation.

Tinctures: Meadowsweet is extracted into alcohol to create a tincture, useful for digestive and joint issues.

Salves-Topical Applications: The herb is infused into creams or ointments to relieve skin irritations and joint pain.

Decoctions: Boiling the roots or leaves of meadowsweet creates a strong decoction for internal use, especially for stomach ailments.

Syrups: Meadowsweet can be simmered with sugar to produce a syrup, easing cold symptoms and sore throats.

Gargles & Mouthwashes: A solution made from meadowsweet extract can be used as a gargle or mouthwash to soothe mouth and throat inflammation.

Powders: Dried and powdered meadowsweet is used in capsules or as a sprinkle on food for digestive health.

Ease to Grow: 2-4, Low Maintenance

Meadowsweet is relatively easy to grow, requiring minimal care. It thrives in moist, fertile soil and partial shade, making it a low-maintenance choice for gardens or wildflower areas.

Milk Thistle

Scientifically known as Silybum Marianum, is a plant recognized for its distinctive purple flowers and white-veined leaves. It is primarily hailed for its seeds, which contain silymarin, a group of compounds said to have antioxidant and anti-inflammatory effects. Traditionally used to treat liver and gallbladder disorders, milk thistle is believed to protect and promote the regeneration of liver cells, combat liver toxins, and improve liver function.

Digestive System

Liver: Milk thistle is renowned for its liver-protective effects, aiding in detoxification processes and liver cell regeneration.

Gallbladder: Promotes bile production and flow, which is essential for digestion and preventing gallstones.

Endocrine System

Pancreas: Milk thistle may help in stabilizing blood sugar levels by improving insulin sensitivity and pancreatic function.

How to Grow Milk Thistle

- **Selecting the Right Variety:** Milk thistle comes primarily in one species, Silybum Marianum. It's best to start with seeds which are readily available online or at health food stores. Look for high-quality, organic seeds to ensure purity and potency.
- **Best Time to Plant Outdoors:** Plant milk thistle seeds in early spring, after the last frost, when the soil is starting to warm up.
- **Spacing Outdoor Plants:** Space plants or seeds about 12 inches apart. Milk thistle can grow tall and wide, so they need room to spread.
- **Container Use and Soil:** Prefers well-draining soil with a neutral to slightly alkaline pH. It can be grown in containers but ensure they are large enough to accommodate the root growth.
- **Sunlight and Location:** Milk thistle needs full sun, at least 6 hours of direct sunlight daily. If using artificial lighting, LED grow lights are suitable.
- **Watering:** Water regularly to keep the soil moist but not waterlogged. Reduce watering once the plants are established.

- **Feeding:** Fertilize lightly in the spring. Milk thistle does not require much feeding; too much can inhibit growth.
- **Pruning and Maintenance:** Snip off dead flowers to prevent the plant from self-seeding excessively. Regularly check for diseased leaves and remove them to keep the plant healthy.
- **Pest and Disease Management:** Watch for common garden pests and treat with organic pesticides if necessary. Milk thistle is relatively disease-resistant but can be affected by fungal infections in overly moist conditions.
- **Overwintering:** In colder climates, milk thistle will die back to the ground and return in spring. In milder climates, it may remain green throughout winter.
- **Propagation:** Milk thistle can self-seed prolifically. Collect seeds in late summer or allow some flowers to go to seed to encourage self-sowing.
- **Harvesting:** Harvest leaves in spring when they are young and tender. Seeds are harvested in late summer when the flower heads turn brown. Dry them for medicinal use.
- **Climate Considerations:** Thrives in warm, dry climates but can adapt to various conditions except for extreme cold or wet areas. Avoid waterlogged soils to prevent root rot.

How to Use Milk Thistle

Herbal Teas or Infusions: Soak milk thistle seeds in hot water to make a detoxifying tea that supports liver health.

Tinctures: Extracted from the seeds, milk thistle tinctures are used to promote liver and gallbladder function.

Salves-Topical Applications: Ground seeds or extract can be mixed into creams for anti-inflammatory and skin-healing.

Decoctions: Boiling the seeds or leaves creates a potent liquid for digestive and liver health.

Powders: Dried and ground seeds are used in capsule form or added to foods for digestive support.

Culinary Uses: Young leaves and shoots can be eaten raw in salads or cooked as greens.

Ease to Grow: 3-5, Low Maintenance

Milk thistle is fairly easy to grow, thriving in sunny locations with well-drained soil. It is resilient, drought-tolerant, and requires minimal maintenance once established. This plant is known for its liver-supportive properties, primarily through the seeds which are used in various medicinal preparations.

Mint

A versatile and aromatic herb, recognized for its refreshing flavor and therapeutic properties. It grows prolifically, making it a popular choice in both culinary and medicinal contexts. Mint leaves are rich in essential oils that have significant health benefits. The aromatic compounds in mint, particularly menthol, contribute to its widespread use in relieving symptoms of various ailments, making it a valuable plant in herbal medicine.

Digestive System

Stomach: Mint soothes the stomach lining, alleviates nausea, and aids in digestion by stimulating the secretion of digestive enzymes and bile.

Respiratory System

Lungs: Mint acts as a decongestant, helping to clear mucus from the lungs and alleviate symptoms of respiratory conditions like asthma and bronchitis.

Nervous System

Brain: Enhances cognitive functions, providing a refreshing and stimulating effect that can improve focus and reduce stress.

Skin and Integumentary System

Skin: The cooling and anti-inflammatory properties of mint help soothe skin irritations, reduce redness, and promote healing.

How to Grow Mint

- **Selecting the Right Variety:** Mint comes in various types, including peppermint and spearmint. Both are beneficial for culinary and medicinal uses. Starting from cuttings or plants is preferable as seeds can be unreliable. You can purchase these at nurseries, garden centers, or online stores.
- **Best Time to Plant Outdoors:** Early spring, after the last frost, is ideal for planting mint. Can also be started indoors around 8-10 weeks before the last frost date.
- **Spacing Outdoor Plants:** Plant mint 18 to 24 inches apart to allow room for growth, as it can spread quickly.

- **Container Use and Soil:** Mint thrives in containers. Use well-draining soil rich in organic matter, with a pH between 6.0 and 7.0.
- **Sunlight and Location:** Mint prefers full sun to partial shade, needing around 4-6 hours of sunlight daily. If growing indoors, use grow lights to supplement light.
- **Watering:** Keep the soil consistently moist but not waterlogged. Water when the top inch of soil feels dry.
- **Feeding:** Apply a balanced, all-purpose liquid fertilizer monthly during the growing season.
- **Pruning and Maintenance:** Regularly snip off dead flowers to encourage bushier growth and prevent the plant from flowering too early and going to seed.
- **Pest and Disease Management:** Watch for aphids and spider mites. Treat with insecticidal soap or neem oil. Prevent fungal diseases by ensuring good air circulation and not overcrowding plants.
- **Overwintering:** In colder climates, mulch over the mint bed to protect roots during winter.
- **Propagation:** Easily propagated by stem cuttings or division in spring or fall.
- **Harvesting:** Harvest leaves as needed, ideally in the morning when essential oil concentrations are highest. Leaves, stems, and flowers are all usable.
- **Climate Considerations:** Mint prefers temperate climates but can adapt to various conditions. It doesn't thrive in extreme heat or cold.

How to Use Mint

Herbal Teas or Infusions: Mint leaves are soaked in hot water to make a refreshing tea, aiding digestion and relieving stomach discomfort.

Tinctures: Mint is concentrated into tinctures to harness its digestive and soothing properties for internal use.

Salves-Topical Applications: Crushed mint leaves are used in creams or ointments for their cooling effect on the skin, reducing irritation and redness.

Compresses: A compress with mint infusion can be applied to areas of the skin to soothe burns or insect bites.

Aromatherapy & Essential Oils: Mint essential oil is used for inhalation to clear nasal passages and for direct application to alleviate headache and nausea.

Herbal Baths: Adding mint leaves to bathwater can provide a soothing and aromatic experience, helping to relieve muscle pain and skin irritation.

Steam Inhalation: Inhaling steam infused with mint leaves can clear the respiratory tract and ease breathing difficulties.

Decoctions: Boiling mint leaves to make a strong decoction can be used for treating gastrointestinal issues.

Syrups: Mint syrup, made by reducing the infusion with sugar, can soothe sore throats and coughs.

Gargles & Mouthwashes: Mint-infused water acts as a mouthwash to freshen breath and reduce oral bacteria.

Powders: Dried and powdered mint leaves can be used for culinary purposes or as a natural deodorant.

Juices: Fresh mint leaves are juiced and added to drinks for flavor and digestive benefits.

Culinary Uses: Mint is widely used in cooking for its flavor, added to dishes, sauces, salads, and drinks.

Ease to Grow: 2-3, Low Maintenance

Mint is incredibly easy to grow, often thriving with minimal care. It prefers well-drained soil and partial to full sunlight. Due to its invasive nature, it's best grown in containers to prevent it from overtaking the garden. Regular watering and occasional pruning will keep it healthy and productive.

Motherwort

(Leonurus Cardiaca) is a perennial plant in the mint family, recognized for its serrated leaves and pink to lilac flowers. Originating from Europe and Asia, it has spread worldwide, valued in traditional medicine for various ailments. Motherwort's name reflects its historical use as a remedy for female reproductive issues, but its applications extend beyond.

Cardiovascular System

Heart: Motherwort is reputed to strengthen and regulate heart function, potentially offering relief from palpitations and tachycardia. It may act as a cardiotonic, improving heart muscle efficiency and stability.

Blood vessels: By promoting vasodilation, motherwort can enhance blood flow and reduce blood pressure, possibly alleviating hypertension and supporting overall cardiovascular health.

Nervous System

Brain: Traditionally used for its anxiolytic properties (reducing anxiety and promoting relaxation), motherwort can calm the mind, reduce anxiety, and alleviate stress, promoting mental well-being. **Nerves:** Its potential sedative effect can soothe nervous agitation, contributing to improved sleep quality and relaxation of the central nervous system.

How to Grow Motherwort

- **Selecting the Right Variety:** Motherwort, primarily Leonurus Cardiaca, is the most beneficial variety. It's preferable to start with seeds, available at online herb and garden stores. Plants or starts can also be used if found.
- **Best Time to Plant Outdoors:** Plant seeds or starts in early spring, after the last frost, to allow the plant to establish before winter.
- **Spacing Outdoor Plants:** Space plants or seeds about 18 to 24 inches apart to ensure adequate air circulation and light penetration.
- **Container Use and Soil:** Motherwort thrives in well-drained soil with a neutral pH. For container planting, use a pot with drainage holes and standard potting mix.
- **Sunlight and Location:** Prefers full sun to partial shade, requiring at least 6 hours of sunlight daily. If using artificial lighting, fluorescent or LED grow lights work well.
- **Watering:** Water regularly to keep the soil consistently moist but not waterlogged, reducing frequency in winter.
- **Feeding:** Apply a balanced, slow-release fertilizer at the beginning of the growing season to support growth.
- **Pruning and Maintenance:** Snip off dead flowers to encourage more blooms and prevent the plant from flowering too early.

- **Pest and Disease Management:** Watch for aphids and powdery mildew. Treat aphids with neem oil and manage mildew by reducing humidity around the plant.
- **Overwintering:** In colder climates, mulch around the base to protect roots from freezing temperatures.
- **Propagation:** Easily propagated by seed or division in spring or autumn.
- **Harvesting:** Leaves and flowering tops can be harvested during blooming. Use them fresh or dried for their medicinal properties.
- **Climate Considerations:** Thrives in temperate climates but can adapt to various conditions, avoiding extremely wet or dry extremes.

How to Use Motherwort

Herbal Teas or Infusions: Soak dried motherwort leaves in hot water for 10-15 minutes to make a calming tea that helps reduce anxiety and improve heart health.

Tinctures: Motherwort is commonly used in tincture form, usually taken in small doses, to help with heart palpitations and menstrual discomfort.

Salves-Topical Applications: Rarely used as a salve, but it can be applied to help heal skin irritations and wounds.

Decoctions: Boil the plant parts to make a strong decoction for use in treating heart conditions and nervous disorders.

Powders: Dried motherwort can be ground into powder and used in capsules for ease of consumption, particularly for cardiovascular and emotional support.

Ease to Grow: 3-5, Low Maintenance

Motherwort is a hardy perennial that grows well in various conditions, making it a low-maintenance choice for gardeners. It adapts easily, and can thrive in partial shade to full sun, making it a reliable plant for medicinal herb gardens.

Mullein

A tall, sturdy herb with soft, velvety leaves and yellow flowers, has been used medicinally for centuries. Known scientifically as Verbascum Thapsus, mullein grows wild in many parts of the world and is prized for its medicinal properties, particularly in herbal medicine. Easily recognizable by its tall stalks that can reach up to 2 meters in height, topped with densely packed yellow flowers. Mullein is known for its ability to soothe respiratory ailments, with a history of use as a remedy for coughs, colds, and bronchial infections. Its leaves and flowers contain compounds that are believed to have anti-inflammatory, antiviral, and antibacterial properties, making it a popular choice for natural treatment of various conditions.

Respiratory System

Lungs: Mullein's expectorant properties help clear mucus, making it beneficial for those suffering from congested coughs and bronchitis. It aids in loosening phlegm and facilitates easier breathing.

Bronchi: Mullein soothes irritated bronchial passages, reduces inflammation, and helps alleviate symptoms of bronchitis and asthma.

Acts as a demulcent (forming a protective layer on the bronchial membranes), and eases irritation.

How to Grow Mullein

- **Selecting the Right Variety:** Mullein has several species, but the most commonly used for medicinal purposes is Verbascum Thapsus. It is typically grown from seeds, which are readily available at nurseries or online stores. Starting with seeds is preferred because it allows for better control over the plant's growing conditions.
- **Best Time to Plant Outdoors:** Sow mullein seeds in late spring or early summer. They require light to germinate, so surface sowing is recommended without covering them with soil.
- **Spacing Outdoor Plants:** Space plants or seeds about 2 feet apart to accommodate their growth, as mullein can grow tall and spread wide.
- **Container Use and Soil:** Mullein grows well in containers using well-draining soil. It prefers slightly alkaline soil but can tolerate a wide range of soil types.
- **Sunlight and Location:** Requires full sun, with at least 6 to 8 hours of direct sunlight daily. If using artificial lighting, fluorescent or LED grow lights are suitable, mimicking natural sunlight conditions.
- **Watering:** Water mullein regularly but allow the soil to dry out between watering to prevent root rot. It is drought-tolerant once established.
- **Feeding:** Mullein does not require frequent fertilization. A light application of a balanced fertilizer at the beginning of the growing season is sufficient.

- **Pruning and Maintenance:** Snip off dead flowers to promote more blooms and prevent the plant from self-seeding excessively.
- **Pest and Disease Management:** Mullein is relatively resistant to pests and diseases. However, watch for signs of rust or leaf spot and treat with fungicides if necessary.
- **Overwintering:** Mullein is biennial (completes its life cycle in two years), so it overwinters naturally. In colder climates, protect the crown of the plant with mulch.
- **Propagation:** Propagate mullein through seed dispersal. The second year of growth will produce seeds that can be collected and sown.
- **Harvesting:** Leaves can be harvested in the first year, while flowers and roots are best harvested in the second year. Use leaves and flowers for herbal remedies; they are beneficial for respiratory health.
- **Climate Considerations:** Thrives in temperate climates and can tolerate cold winters. Avoid excessively wet or humid conditions as they may lead to root diseases.

How to Use Mullein

Herbal Teas or Infusions: Leaves or flowers of mullein are soaked in hot water to make a tea, beneficial for respiratory ailments like cough and congestion.

Tinctures: Both leaves and flowers can be used to make a tincture, aiding in respiratory and inflammatory conditions.

Salves-Topical Applications: A salve made from mullein leaves can be applied to the skin to soothe irritation, burns, and hemorrhoids.

Poultices: Fresh or dried mullein leaves are moistened and applied directly to the skin to reduce inflammation and pain.

Compresses: Mullein leaves infused in water can be used as a compress to treat skin inflammations and infections.

Decoctions: Boiling the leaves or roots to make a strong tea helps in treating gastrointestinal issues and internal infections.

Syrups: Mullein flowers and leaves can be made into a syrup, often used for coughs and sore throats.

Gargles & Mouthwashes: A tea made from the leaves or flowers can be used as a gargle or mouthwash to alleviate throat irritations.

Ease to Grow: 2-4, Low Maintenance

Mullein is a hardy plant that grows well in poor soil conditions and requires minimal care.

Neem

Known scientifically as Azadirachta Indica, is a tree native to the Indian subcontinent. Esteemed for its myriad uses in traditional medicine, neem leaves, bark, and oil possess antibacterial, antifungal, and anti-inflammatory properties. It is often called the "village pharmacy" because every part of the tree can be used for health and wellness.

Digestive System

Stomach: Neem can reduce ulcers and acidity, helping to maintain the stomach lining's integrity and aiding in the prevention of gastrointestinal disorders.

Intestines: It acts against intestinal parasites, enhancing digestive health and nutrient absorption.

Immune System

General Immunity: Neem boosts the immune system by increasing the body's response to infections, reducing susceptibility to various pathogens.

Skin and Integumentary System

Skin: Neem is used topically to treat acne and eczema, promoting healing and reducing inflammation. It enhances the skin's barrier function and helps in controlling bacterial infections.

How to Grow Neem

- **Selecting the Right Variety:** Neem trees are generally of one main variety, known for their medicinal properties. It is preferable to start with seeds or young plants, which can be purchased from specialized nurseries or online stores focusing on medicinal or tropical plants.
- **Best Time to Plant Outdoors:** The ideal time to plant neem trees is at the beginning of the rainy season or in early spring to ensure they get plenty of water to establish their roots.
- **Spacing Outdoor Plants:** Plants should be spaced at least 20 feet apart to allow room for growth, as neem trees can grow large.
- **Container Use and Soil:** Neem trees can grow in pots initially but prefer to be planted in the ground. They need well-draining soil, rich in organic matter. For container

growth, use a large pot with plenty of room for root development.

- **Sunlight and Location:** Neem trees require full sunlight, at least six hours of direct sunlight daily. If using artificial lighting, LED grow lights can provide the full spectrum they need.
- **Watering:** Water young plants regularly to establish roots, then water moderately. Neem trees are drought-resistant but perform best with consistent moisture.
- **Feeding:** Apply a balanced, slow-release fertilizer during the growing season to support leaf and branch development.
- **Pruning and Maintenance:** Regularly snip off dead flowers and prune to shape the tree and encourage growth. Remove any dead or diseased branches to maintain plant health.
- **Pest and Disease Management:** Neem trees are generally resistant to pests and diseases. However, watch for common issues like leaf spot or root rot and treat with appropriate organic methods.
- **Overwintering:** In cooler climates, neem trees should be protected from frost. They can be grown in large containers and moved indoors during colder months.
- **Propagation:** Propagate through seeds, cuttings, or root division in spring or early summer. Seeds have a short viability period and should be planted soon after harvesting.
- **Harvesting:** Leaves, bark, seeds, and flowers can be harvested. Leaves and seeds are commonly used in herbal remedies. Harvest leaves any time, preferably in the morning, and seeds after the fruit ripens.
- **Climate Considerations:** Neem trees thrive in tropical to subtropical climates, with temps between 69-95°F. They can tolerate brief cold spells but need protection from frost.

How to Use Neem

Herbal Teas or Infusions: Neem leaves are soaked in hot water to create a bitter tea, often consumed for its health benefits, particularly for skin and digestive health.

Tinctures: A tincture is made from neem leaves or bark, used for its concentrated medicinal properties, especially in treating skin conditions and detoxifying the body.

Salves-Topical Applications: Neem oil, extracted from the seeds, is incorporated into creams or ointments for treating skin infections, eczema, and acne.

Decoctions: Boiling neem bark or leaves in water makes a decoction used to wash wounds or treat dental and gum diseases.

Powders: Dried neem leaves can be ground into powder, and used both internally for digestive health and externally as a paste for skin issues.

Ease to Grow: 4-6, Medium Maintenance

Neem trees are reasonably straightforward to cultivate in the right climate, requiring a warm environment and minimal maintenance once established. They are resilient to pests and diseases, which contributes to their medium maintenance level

---

Nettle

Scientifically known as Urtica Dioica, is a perennial herb renowned for its stinging hairs on the leaves and stems. This plant is highly valued in herbal medicine, offering a range of health benefits due to its rich content of vitamins, minerals, and potent phytochemicals. Nettle has been traditionally used to treat various ailments, demonstrating its versatility in herbal therapy.

Digestive System

Stomach: Nettle aids in digestion by stimulating gastric secretions and reducing inflammation in the GI tract.

Intestines: Supports intestinal health by promoting the growth of beneficial gut flora and enhancing nutrient absorption.

Respiratory System

Lungs: Nettle acts as an expectorant, helping to alleviate symptoms of respiratory conditions like asthma and hay fever by reducing inflammation and mucus production.

Urinary System

Kidneys: Nettle is a natural diuretic, increasing urine production and helping to flush out toxins from the kidneys, which can prevent urinary tract infections and kidney stones.

Musculoskeletal System

Joints: Its anti-inflammatory properties are beneficial in treating painful conditions like arthritis and gout, reducing swelling and pain in the joints.

How to Grow Nettle

- **Selecting the Right Variety:** Nettle has several varieties, but Urtica Dioica is the most commonly used for medicinal purposes. It can be started from seeds or starts, with seeds readily available online or at local nurseries.
- **Best Time to Plant Outdoors:** Early spring is ideal for planting nettle outdoors, as the plant prefers cooler temperatures to establish its roots.
- **Spacing Outdoor Plants:** Space plants or seeds about 12 inches apart to allow for adequate growth and air circulation.
- **Container Use and Soil:** Nettle thrives in rich, moist, well-draining soil with a pH of 6 to 7. It can grow in containers, but ensure they are deep enough to accommodate the long roots.
- **Sunlight and Location:** Prefers partial shade but can tolerate full sun; requires at least 4-6 hours of sunlight daily. In very hot climates, protect from intense afternoon sun.
- **Watering:** Keep the soil consistently moist, especially during dry periods. Nettle does not like to dry out completely.
- **Feeding:** Apply a balanced liquid fertilizer every 4-6 weeks during the growing season to support robust growth.
- **Pruning and Maintenance:** Regularly snip off dead flowers to encourage more leaf growth and prevent the plant from flowering too early.
- **Pest and Disease Management:** Nettle is generally hardy but watch for common garden pests like aphids. Treat with organic pesticides if necessary.
- **Overwintering:** In colder zones, mulch around the base to protect roots from freezing. In warmer climates, nettle may remain green throughout winter.

- **Propagation:** Easily propagated by root division in autumn or spring. Seeds can self-sow, leading to natural spreading.
- **Harvesting:** Harvest leaves before the plant flowers, typically in late spring to early summer. Leaves, stems, and roots can be used for their medicinal properties. Wear gloves to avoid stings.
- **Climate Considerations:** Nettle is adaptable but thrives best in temperatures between 35°F and 85°F. It can tolerate frost and prefers climates where it can experience a dormant winter period.

How to Use Nettle

Herbal Teas or Infusions: Nettle leaves are soaked in hot water to make a herbal tea, known for its rich mineral content and anti-inflammatory properties.

Tinctures: Made from the leaves or roots, nettle tinctures are used to alleviate allergy symptoms and support urinary health.

Salves-Topical Applications: Nettle is infused into salves to soothe skin irritations, eczema, and joint pain.

Compresses: Soaked leaves are applied directly to the skin to relieve arthritis pain and skin issues.

Herbal Baths: Nettle can be added to bathwater to help with skin conditions and improve circulation.

Steam Inhalation: Inhaling steam from boiled nettle leaves can alleviate respiratory conditions.

Decoctions: Boiling the roots or leaves to concentrate its compounds, used for urinary and joint support.

Syrups: Nettle syrup, often combined with other herbs, is used to relieve cough and cold symptoms.

Gargles & Mouthwashes: A solution made from nettle is used to treat sore throats and oral inflammation.

Powders: Dried and powdered nettle leaves are used in supplements for nutritional benefits.

Juices: Fresh nettle leaves are juiced and consumed for detoxification and nutritional benefits.

Culinary Uses: Young nettle leaves are cooked and eaten as a nutritious green, similar to spinach.

Ease to Grow: 2-4, Low Maintenance

Nettle is straightforward to cultivate, thriving in various environments, from full sun to partial shade, and requiring minimal maintenance. Adaptable to different soil types, it's known for its hardiness and ability to self-seed, making it a resilient plant suitable for novice gardeners.

Nutmeg

Derived from the seed of the Myristica Fragrans tree, it is renowned for its aromatic and culinary applications. Beyond its culinary uses, nutmeg has significant medicinal properties. It contains compounds like myristicin and eugenol, which have antioxidant, anti-inflammatory, and antimicrobial effects. Traditionally, nutmeg has been used to treat various ailments, ranging from digestive issues to pain relief and insomnia.

Digestive System

Stomach: Nutmeg aids digestion, reduces flatulence, and alleviates nausea, thanks to its carminative properties (ability to relieve gastrointestinal discomfort, particularly bloating, gas, and indigestion).

Digestion Aid: Promotes healthy digestion by stimulating the secretion of digestive enzymes, which helps break down food more effectively. This can lead to reduced bloating and discomfort after meals.

Flatulence Reduction: Nutmeg helps reduce flatulence or excessive gas in the digestive tract, and can help ease discomfort associated with gas buildup.

Nausea Alleviation: Nutmeg is often used as a natural remedy to alleviate nausea and vomiting. Its calming effects on the stomach can provide relief from feelings of queasiness.

How to Grow Nutmeg

- **Selecting the Right Variety:** Nutmeg comes from the Myristica Fragrans tree; no varieties as such, but ensure you get healthy seeds. Start with seeds directly sourced from a reputable supplier. These are available online or at specialty garden stores that sell exotic or tropical plant seeds.
- **Best Time to Plant Outdoors:** Plant nutmeg seeds in spring or early summer when temperatures are consistently above 60°F. They need a warm climate to thrive.
- **Spacing Outdoor Plants:** Space nutmeg trees about 20 to 30 feet apart as they grow large. Ensure ample space for root and canopy expansion.
- **Container Use and Soil:** Use large containers with well-draining soil rich in organic matter. A mix of potting soil,

compost, and sand works well for good drainage and nutrient provision.

- **Sunlight and Location:** Nutmeg trees require partial to full sunlight, about 6-8 hours daily. In areas with intense heat, provide some afternoon shade.
- **Watering:** Water regularly to keep the soil moist but not waterlogged. Nutmeg trees like humidity and consistent moisture.
- **Feeding:** Fertilize with a balanced, slow-release fertilizer during the growing season to support growth and fruit production.
- **Pruning and Maintenance:** Snip off dead flowers to encourage more growth. Regular pruning helps maintain shape and health, removing any diseased or overgrown branches.
- **Pest and Disease Management:** Watch for signs like wilted leaves or stunted growth, indicating pest or disease issues. Treat with organic pesticides or fungicides as needed.
- **Overwintering:** In cooler climates, nutmeg trees must be grown in containers and brought indoors or protected during winter, as they cannot tolerate temperatures below 50°F.
- **Propagation:** Propagated through seeds. Plant fresh seeds as they lose viability quickly.
- **Harvesting:** Harvest the nutmeg fruit when it splits open, revealing the red aril (mace) and the seed (nutmeg) inside. Dry both mace and nutmeg in the sun before using or storing.
- **Climate Considerations:** Best grown in warm, tropical climates with temperatures consistently between 70°F and 90°F. They require high humidity and well-distributed rainfall throughout the year.

How to Use Nutmeg

Herbal Teas or Infusions: Ground nutmeg is soaked in hot water to create a flavorful tea, often used for its calming and digestive benefits.

Tinctures: Nutmeg is macerated in alcohol to extract its therapeutic properties, creating a tincture used in small doses for its medicinal effects.

Salves-Topical Applications: Nutmeg oil is blended with carrier oils to make creams or ointments for pain relief and to soothe skin conditions.

Aromatherapy & Essential Oils: Nutmeg essential oil is used in aromatherapy diffusers or applied topically when diluted with a carrier oil, for pain relief and to promote relaxation.

Culinary Uses: Used widely in cooking and baking, grated or ground, to add flavor to dishes like pies, sauces, and beverages.

Ease to Grow: 8-10, High Maintenance-Expert

Nutmeg trees require a tropical climate, consistent moisture, and cannot tolerate cold. Growing nutmeg is a long-term commitment as it takes years for the trees to mature and produce fruit. The process is complex, needing specific climatic conditions, making it challenging to grow outside its native environment.

Oregano

A perennial herb famous for its aromatic leaves, is a staple in Mediterranean cuisine and renowned for its potent antioxidants and anti-inflammatory properties. Thriving in warm climates, oregano contains compounds like thymol and carvacrol, which contribute to its medicinal benefits. Traditionally, oregano has been used to treat various ailments, adding to its antibacterial, antiviral, and antifungal effects.

Respiratory System

Lungs: Oregano's compounds help soothe coughs and can alleviate respiratory tract infections by acting as an expectorant to clear mucus.
Bronchi: Its antispasmodic properties aid in relieving bronchial spasms, making it beneficial for asthma and bronchitis sufferers.

Digestive System

Stomach: Oregano stimulates appetite and aids digestion by increasing bile flow and aiding in the breakdown of food.
Intestines: Has antimicrobial properties that combat intestinal parasites and can alleviate gastrointestinal infections.

Immune System

General Immunity: The antioxidants in oregano strengthen the immune system, helping the body fight against infections and diseases more effectively.

Skin and Integumentary System

Skin: Its antiseptic and anti-inflammatory qualities make oregano oil useful in treating skin infections, irritations, and inflammatory conditions like acne and eczema.

How to Grow Oregano

- **Selecting the Right Variety:** Common varieties of oregano include Greek, Italian, and Golden. Greek oregano is most flavorful; ideal for culinary use. Start with seeds or young plants, available at nurseries or online garden shops.

- **Best Time to Plant Outdoors:** Plant oregano in spring after the last frost, typically in late March to April, to ensure a warm growing environment.

- **Spacing Outdoor Plants:** Space oregano plants or seeds about 8 to 10 inches apart to allow for growth and airflow, reducing the risk of disease.

- **Container Use and Soil:** Oregano thrives in well-draining soil with a pH of 6.0 to 7.0. In containers, use a mix of potting soil and perlite or sand for improved drainage.

- **Sunlight and Location:** Oregano requires full sun, meaning at least 6 to 8 hours of direct sunlight daily. For indoor growth, use grow lights to provide adequate light.

- **Watering:** Water oregano when the soil feels dry to the touch. Overwatering can lead to root rot, so ensure good drainage.

- **Feeding:** Fertilize oregano sparingly; too much fertilizer can diminish its flavor. A light application of organic fertilizer in the spring is sufficient.

- **Pruning and Maintenance:** Regularly snip off dead flowers to encourage bushier growth and prevent the plant from flowering too early.
- **Pest and Disease Management:** Watch for aphids and spider mites. Treat with neem oil or insecticidal soap. Root rot appears as wilted, yellow leaves; improve drainage and reduce watering to manage.
- **Overwintering:** In cooler climates, mulch around the base to protect roots or bring containers indoors during winter.
- **Propagation:** Propagate by cuttings or division in early summer. Cuttings root easily in water or soil.
- **Harvesting:** Harvest leaves before the plant flowers for the best flavor. Use fresh, or dry them for later use.
- **Climate Considerations:** Oregano prefers warm climates with temperatures between 70°F and 80°F. It can tolerate down to 50°F but will not survive freezing temperatures.

How to Use Oregano

Herbal Teas or Infusions: Oregano leaves are soaked in hot water for several minutes to make a herbal tea known for its antioxidant properties and soothing effects on the digestive system.

Tinctures: Oregano leaves are steeped in alcohol to extract their essential oils, creating a potent tincture for internal or topical use.

Salves-Topical Applications: Oregano oil is mixed with a carrier oil or beeswax to make salves or ointments for treating skin infections and irritations.

Poultices: Crushed oregano leaves can be applied directly to the skin to relieve inflammation and pain.

Compresses: A cloth soaked in oregano-infused water is applied to the skin to soothe and reduce discomfort.

Aromatherapy & Essential Oils: Oregano essential oil is used in diffusers or inhaled directly for respiratory relief and to boost immunity.

Herbal Baths: Adding oregano leaves to bathwater helps in relaxing muscles and improving skin health.

Steam Inhalation: Inhaling steam infused with oregano leaves can clear nasal passages and relieve respiratory conditions.

Decoctions: Boiling oregano leaves to concentrate their active compounds creates a strong liquid used for medicinal purposes.

Syrups: Oregano leaves are often boiled with sugar to make a syrup, used to soothe coughs and sore throats.

Gargles & Mouthwashes: A solution made from oregano leaves can be used as a mouthwash or gargle to treat oral infections and sore throats.

Powders: Dried and ground oregano leaves are used as a powder for culinary and medicinal purposes.

Juices: Fresh oregano leaves are juiced and consumed for their health benefits.

Culinary Uses: Oregano is widely used as a seasoning in Mediterranean cuisine, adding flavor to dishes while providing several health benefits.

Ease to Grow: 2-3, Low Maintenance

Oregano is a hardy herb that's easy to grow, requiring minimal maintenance. It thrives in well-draining soil and full sunlight, making it an excellent choice for beginner gardeners. Its resilience to pests and diseases adds to its appeal as a low-maintenance herb.

Parsley

A versatile culinary herb known for its vibrant taste and nutritional benefits. It belongs to the Apiaceae family and is native to the Mediterranean region. Parsley is rich in vitamins A, C, and K, and minerals like iron and potassium. It has been used traditionally for its diuretic, digestive, and anti-inflammatory properties. Parsley's high antioxidant content supports overall health and wellness.

Digestive System

Stomach: Parsley aids in digestion by stimulating digestive enzymes and relieving gas and bloating.

Intestines: Acts as a mild laxative, helping to ease constipation and regulate bowel movements.

Urinary System

Kidneys: As a natural diuretic, parsley promotes urine production and flow, aiding in the removal of toxins from the body.

Cardiovascular System

Blood Vessels: The high vitamin C and antioxidant content in parsley helps strengthen blood vessels and reduce the risk of atherosclerosis (plaque build-up).

Immune System

General Immunity: Parsley's vitamin C content boosts the immune system, helping the body to fight off infections and diseases.

Endocrine System

Pancreas: Parsley may help regulate blood sugar levels, supporting pancreatic health and function.

How to Grow Parsley

- **Selecting the Right Variety:** Parsley comes in two main types, flat-leaf (Italian) and curly-leaf. Flat-leaf parsley is more flavorful and used in cooking, while curly-leaf is often used as a garnish. Both varieties can be grown from seeds or starts, with seeds being more commonly used. Seeds are available in garden centers or online.

- **Best Time to Plant Outdoors:** The best time to plant parsley outdoors is in early spring, once the risk of frost has passed. In warmer climates, it can also be planted in the fall for winter harvest.

- **Spacing Outdoor Plants:** Plant parsley seeds or starts about 6 to 8 inches apart in rows. This spacing allows ample room for growth and air circulation.

- **Container Use and Soil:** Parsley thrives in containers with well-draining soil. Use a potting mix designed for vegetables or herbs. Ensure the container has drainage holes to prevent waterlogging.

- **Sunlight and Location:** Parsley prefers full sun but can tolerate partial shade. It needs around 6 to 8 hours of sunlight daily. In hot climates, afternoon shade can prevent it from flowering too early.

- **Watering:** Keep the soil consistently moist but not waterlogged. Water parsley deeply once or twice a week, depending on weather conditions.
- **Feeding:** Apply a balanced liquid fertilizer every 4 to 6 weeks during the growing season to support healthy growth.
- **Pruning and Maintenance:** Snip off dead flowers to encourage bushier growth and prevent the plant from going to seed early.
- **Pest and Disease Management:** Watch for common pests like aphids and treat with insecticidal soap if necessary. Root rot can occur in overly wet soil, so ensure good drainage.
- **Overwintering:** In colder regions, mulch around the parsley plants to protect them through the winter.
- **Propagation:** Parsley can be propagated from seeds or by dividing mature plants. It's biennial, so seed saving can be done in the second year.
- **Harvesting:** Harvest parsley leaves as needed, starting from the outer portions of the plant. The best flavor is achieved when harvested in the morning.
- **Climate Considerations:** Parsley grows best in temperate climates with temperatures between 50 and 70°F. It can tolerate light frost but not prolonged cold or extreme heat.

How to Use Parsley

Herbal Teas or Infusions: Parsley leaves can be soaked in hot water to make an herbal tea known for its diuretic properties and support of kidney health.

Tinctures: A parsley tincture is used for its diuretic effects and to support urinary tract health.

Decoctions: Can be used in a decoction to help with digestive issues and as a natural diuretic.

Gargles & Mouthwashes: Parsley can be used in a mouthwash for its antimicrobial properties, helping to freshen breath.

Powders: Dried parsley can be powdered and used as a spice or for its health benefits in capsule form.

Juices: Fresh parsley can be juiced and consumed for its high vitamin and mineral content, particularly for vitamins A, C, and K.

Culinary Uses: Widely used in cooking for flavoring dishes, including soups, sauces, and salads. It's also known for its ability to neutralize bad breath.

Ease to Grow: 2-4, Low Maintenance

Parsley is a robust herb that is relatively easy to grow, requiring basic gardening care. It thrives in well-drained soil with ample sunlight and regular watering. Being low maintenance, it's suitable for gardeners of all levels, offering both culinary and medicinal benefits.

Passionflower

Also known as Passiflora, is renowned for its striking flowers and medicinal properties. It's primarily recognized for its calming and sleep-inducing effects, making it a popular remedy for anxiety and insomnia. Passionflower acts as a mild sedative, soothing the nervous system and aiding in relaxation. It's often used in herbal teas, extracts, and supplements for its therapeutic benefits.

Nervous System

Brain: Passionflower can enhance gamma-aminobutyric acid (GABA) levels in the brain, helping to reduce anxiety and promote relaxation.

Nerves: It possesses nerve-soothing properties that help alleviate nerve pain and symptoms of nervous disorder.

How to Grow Passionflower

- **Selecting the Right Variety:** Passionflower has many varieties; Passiflora Incarnata is most commonly used for medicinal purposes. It's preferable to start with seedlings or cuttings, as seeds can be slow to germinate. You can purchase these from nurseries, garden centers, or online stores specializing in medicinal plants.
- **Best Time to Plant Outdoors:** Spring is the best time to plant Passionflower outdoors, after the last frost, to give the plant a full growing season to establish.
- **Spacing Outdoor Plants:** Space plants at least 6 to 8 feet apart, as Passionflower vines can grow quite large and need room to spread.
- **Container Use and Soil:** Passionflower can be grown in containers with well-draining soil mixed with compost. For outdoor planting, use rich, loamy soil with good drainage.
- **Sunlight and Location:** Requires full sun to partial shade, with at least 4-6 hours of sunlight daily. In regions with very hot summers, some afternoon shade is beneficial. For artificial lighting, use grow lights positioned 12-24 inches above the plants.
- **Watering:** Keep the soil consistently moist but not waterlogged. Watering should be more frequent during dry periods.

- **Feeding:** Apply a balanced, slow-release fertilizer at the beginning of the growing season to support growth.
- **Pruning and Maintenance:** Regularly snip off dead flowers to encourage more blooms. Prune in early spring to control growth and shape the plant.
- **Pest and Disease Management:** Watch for common pests like aphids and spider mites. Treat with organic insecticidal soap or neem oil. Fungal diseases can occur in overly moist conditions; ensure good air circulation and use fungicides if necessary.
- **Overwintering:** In colder climates, mulch around the base or bring containers indoors to protect from freezing temperatures.
- **Propagation:** Propagate by seed, cuttings, or layering in early summer. Cuttings root easily in moist soil or water.
- **Harvesting:** Harvest leaves and flowers in the morning after dew has dried but before the sun is at its peak, typically in the second year. Use them fresh or dry them for later use.
- **Climate Considerations:** Thrives in warm, temperate climates but can be grown in a variety of regions. Prefers temperatures between 60 and 80 degrees Fahrenheit and does not tolerate extreme cold very well.

How to Use Passionflower

Herbal Teas or Infusions: Passionflower leaves and flowers are soaked in hot water to create a calming tea, often used to alleviate anxiety and improve sleep quality.

Tinctures: A concentrated liquid extract is made from passionflower, used for its sedative and anxiolytic effects, typically administered in small doses.

Salves-Topical Applications: The extracts of passionflower are used for creams or ointments for their soothing properties on skin irritations and inflammations.

Compresses: Infused passionflower tea or decoction is used in compresses to relieve skin conditions or aches.

Aromatherapy & Essential Oils: While not commonly distilled into essential oils, the scent of fresh passionflower can be used for relaxation in aromatherapy practices.

Decoctions: A stronger, boiled extract of passionflower is made for more potent therapeutic use, especially for digestive and sleep issues.

Syrups: Passionflower extract is mixed into syrups for ease of use, often to help with insomnia or nervous disorders.

Powders: Dried Passionflower can be ground into a powder and used in capsules or mixed into beverages for medicinal use.

Ease to Grow: 3-5, Low to Medium Maintenance

Passionflower is relatively easy to grow, requiring minimal care once established. It prefers well-drained soil and a sunny location but tolerates partial shade. Being a vigorous vine, it needs space to spread and a structure to climb. It's resilient against pests and diseases, making it a low to medium maintenance plant.

Peppermint

A perennial herb, is renowned for its aromatic leaves and is widely used in both culinary and medicinal applications. It contains menthol, which provides its cooling sensation and characteristic minty aroma. Peppermint has been used historically to alleviate various ailments, enhancing its value in traditional and herbal medicine.

Digestive System

Stomach: Peppermint relaxes the stomach muscles, helps relieve symptoms of indigestion, bloating, and gas, and can reduce nausea.

Intestines: It eases irritable bowel syndrome symptoms by relaxing the intestinal tract and reducing intestinal spasms.

Nervous System

Brain: Peppermint enhances cognitive functions and helps in relieving headaches, including migraines, by improving blood flow and reducing pain.

Respiratory System

Lungs: The menthol in peppermint acts as an expectorant, aiding in the clearing of mucus from the lungs and providing relief from coughs, colds, and sinusitis.

Cardiovascular System

Circulation: Peppermint can invigorate blood flow, potentially helping to improve circulation and relieve symptoms of cold hands and feet.

Immune System

General Immunity: Its antimicrobial and antiviral properties strengthen the body's defense mechanisms against infections.

Skin and Integumentary System

Skin: Peppermint oil is used topically to cool and soothe irritated skin, relieve itching, and reduce redness and inflammation.

How to Grow Peppermint

- **Selecting the Right Variety:** Peppermint does not grow true to seed, so it's best to purchase plants or obtain cuttings from a trusted source. Varieties like 'Black Mitcham' are popular for their strong flavor. You can find plants at nurseries, garden centers, or online.

- **Best Time to Plant Outdoors:** Early spring, after the last frost, is ideal for planting peppermint. It gives the plant ample time to establish before summer.

- **Spacing Outdoor Plants:** Plant peppermint 18 to 24 inches apart to allow room for spreading. It grows vigorously and can become invasive.

- **Container Use and Soil:** Grow in containers to control spread. Use well-draining soil rich in organic matter. Pots should have good drainage holes.

- **Sunlight and Location:** Peppermint prefers partial shade to full sun, needing about 4-6 hours of sunlight daily. It can tolerate indirect light and is suitable for indoor growth under grow lights.

- **Watering:** Keep the soil consistently moist but not waterlogged. Peppermint thrives with regular watering, especially during dry periods.

- **Feeding:** Fertilize lightly in the spring and mid-summer with a balanced, all-purpose fertilizer to support growth.

- **Pruning and Maintenance:** Regularly snip off dead flowers to promote bushy growth and prevent the plant from flowering too early, which can reduce leaf quality.
- **Pest and Disease Management:** Watch for common pests like spider mites and aphids. Treat with neem oil or insecticidal soap. Root rot can occur in overly wet soil, so ensure good drainage.
- **Overwintering:** In colder climates, mulch around the base to protect roots from freezing temperatures. Container plants can be moved indoors.
- **Propagation:** Easily propagated by division or cuttings in the spring or fall. Cuttings can be rooted in water or directly in soil.
- **Harvesting:** Harvest leaves just before the plant flowers for the best flavor. Leaves can be used fresh or dried for later use. Collect leaves in the morning after dew has evaporated.
- **Climate Considerations:** Peppermint thrives in cool, moist conditions and is tolerant of a wide range of temperatures. It may struggle in excessively hot and dry climates if not provided with sufficient water.

How to Use Peppermint

Herbal Teas or Infusions: Soak peppermint leaves in boiling water for 5 to 10 minutes to make a refreshing tea that aids digestion and relieves stomach discomfort.

Tinctures: Peppermint leaves are soaked in alcohol to extract their active ingredients, creating a tincture that can be used for digestive issues.

Salves-Topical Applications: Crushed peppermint leaves can be mixed into creams or ointments to relieve muscle pain and itching.

Compresses: A cloth soaked in peppermint tea can be applied to the skin to soothe headaches or skin irritation.

Aromatherapy & Essential Oils: Peppermint oil is used in diffusers or applied topically (diluted) to relieve stress, boost energy, and help with respiratory issues.

Herbal Baths: Adding peppermint leaves to bathwater can create a soothing soak that relieves skin irritations and muscle pain.

Steam Inhalation: Inhaling steam infused with peppermint oil can clear nasal passages and relieve respiratory conditions.

Decoctions: Boiling peppermint leaves in water makes a strong decoction that can help with coughs and colds.

Syrups: Peppermint leaves are often simmered with sugar and water to make a syrup that soothes sore throats.

Gargles & Mouthwashes: A solution made from peppermint infusion is used as a mouthwash to freshen breath and kill bacteria.

Powders: Dried and powdered peppermint leaves are used in capsules or as a seasoning.

Juices: Peppermint leaves are juiced and consumed for their digestive and nutritional benefits.

Culinary Uses: Fresh or dried peppermint leaves are used in cooking for their aromatic flavor, particularly in sauces, teas, and desserts.

Ease to Grow: 2-4, Low Maintenance

Peppermint is quite easy to grow, thriving in partial shade to full sun with moist, well-drained soil. It's a vigorous plant that spreads quickly, so containment is often the main challenge. Its hardiness and low maintenance requirements make it a good choice for beginner gardeners.

Perilla

Also known as Perilla Frutescens, is an herb belonging to the mint family and is widely recognized for its culinary and medicinal properties. It is commonly used in Asian cuisine and is known for its distinct, aromatic flavor. Perilla leaves contain a variety of nutrients, including vitamins, minerals, and essential oils. In traditional medicine, perilla is used to treat a range of ailments due to its anti-inflammatory, antioxidant, and antiallergic properties.

Respiratory System

Lungs: Perilla helps alleviate asthma symptoms and coughs by reducing inflammation and acting as an expectorant to clear respiratory passages.

Immune System

General Immunity: Perilla boosts the immune system due to its antioxidant properties, helping to protect the body against pathogens and reduce inflammation.

Digestive System

Stomach: Perilla is known to soothe the stomach, relieve indigestion, and reduce bloating by promoting healthy digestion and alleviating gastrointestinal discomfort.

Cardiovascular System

Blood Vessels: Perilla oil, rich in alpha-linolenic acid, contributes to cardiovascular health by helping to lower blood cholesterol levels and maintain healthy blood pressure.

How to Grow Perilla

- **Selecting the Right Variety:** Perilla comes in varieties like Perilla Frutescens (green perilla) and Perilla Frutescens var. crispa (purple perilla), both valued for their unique flavors and health benefits. Seeds are the preferred starting method, widely available in online stores or garden centers, offering an easy and effective way to grow perilla.
- **Best Time to Plant Outdoors:** Plant perilla seeds outdoors in spring, after the last frost, when the soil temperature has warmed up sufficiently.
- **Spacing Outdoor Plants:** Space plants or seeds about 10 to 12 inches apart to ensure adequate air circulation and room for growth.
- **Container Use and Soil:** Perilla grows well in containers with well-draining soil. A standard potting mix enriched with compost works well for both container and garden planting.
- **Sunlight and Location:** Perilla needs full sun to partial shade, requiring at least 6 hours of sunlight daily. If growing indoors, provide bright, indirect light or use a grow light for sufficient exposure.
- **Watering:** Keep the soil consistently moist but not waterlogged. Water perilla plants when the top inch of soil feels dry to the touch.
- **Feeding:** Feed perilla with a balanced liquid fertilizer once a month during the growing season to support its vigorous growth.

- **Pruning and Maintenance:** Snip off dead flowers to promote bushier growth and prevent the plant from flowering too early, which can lead to a decline in leaf quality.
- **Pest and Disease Management:** Perilla is relatively pest-resistant but can be affected by aphids and spider mites. Use insecticidal soap or neem oil as a treatment. Watch for fungal diseases and improve air circulation or reduce leaf wetness to manage them.
- **Overwintering:** In cooler climates, perilla is treated as an annual. It can reseed itself or be propagated indoors to ensure a supply for the next season.
- **Propagation:** Easily propagated by seeds; you can also take stem cuttings in late summer for indoor growth over winter.
- **Harvesting:** Leaves can be harvested throughout the growing season as needed. They are the most commonly used part, harvested before the plant flowers for the best flavor and nutritional content.
- **Climate Considerations:** Perilla prefers climates with warm summers and mild winters. It can grow in various environments but thrives in areas with well-defined seasons and adequate rainfall or irrigation.

How to Use Perilla

Herbal Teas or Infusions: Perilla leaves can be soaked in hot water to make an herbal tea, which is consumed for its potential respiratory benefits and to alleviate symptoms of colds and flu.

Tinctures: Perilla leaves are used in tinctures to extract their beneficial compounds, aiding in respiratory health and immune support.

Decoctions: A decoction of perilla leaves can be prepared by boiling them in water, used to help with symptoms of nausea and indigestion.

Juices: The leaves of perilla are juiced to harness their rich nutrient profile, including antioxidants, which can support overall health and well-being.

Culinary Uses: Perilla leaves are commonly used in Asian cuisine, adding a unique flavor to dishes like salads, soups, and marinades, and are known for their health-promoting properties.

Ease to Grow: 2-3, Low Maintenance

Perilla is considered low maintenance and easy to grow, thriving in a range of soil types and conditions. Prefers full sun to partial shade and requires regular watering without being waterlogged. Perilla is an excellent choice for beginner gardeners.

Plantain

Often regarded as a common weed, it is actually a versatile and beneficial herb. This hardy plant, characterized by its broad, ribbed leaves and fibrous stalks, thrives in disturbed soils worldwide. Plantain is known for its healing properties, particularly in wound care and inflammation reduction. It's packed with nutrients, including vitamins A and C, calcium, and iron, making it a valuable addition to herbal remedies.

Respiratory System

Lungs: Plantain acts as an expectorant, facilitating the expulsion of mucus and easing coughs.

Skin and Integumentary System

Wounds and Skin Irritations: Plantain is used topically for its antibacterial and anti-inflammatory properties, speeding up the healing of cuts, bites, and rashes.

Digestive System

Digestive Tract: The mucilage in plantain provides a soothing effect on the digestive tract, helping to treat ulcers and acid reflux.

Immune System

General Immunity: Plantain enhances your immune response, aiding in the body's defense against infections.

How to Grow Plantain

- **Selecting the Right Variety:** Common plantain (Plantago Major) and ribwort plantain (Plantago Lanceolata) are the most beneficial varieties. Both can be grown from seeds, which are available at nurseries or online garden stores.
- **Best Time to Plant Outdoors:** Early spring is ideal for planting outdoors, as the seeds require cool temperatures to germinate.
- **Spacing Outdoor Plants:** Seeds should be sown directly into the ground, spaced about 6 inches apart, as plantain doesn't require much room to grow.

- **Container Use and Soil:** Plantain can thrive in pots using well-draining soil. It's adaptable but prefers slightly moist, fertile soil with a neutral to slightly acidic pH.
- **Sunlight and Location:** Prefers full sun to partial shade. If growing indoors, use grow lights to provide at least six hours of light daily.
- **Watering:** Keep the soil consistently moist but not waterlogged. Plantain is drought-tolerant once established but benefits from regular watering.
- **Feeding:** Fertilize sparingly, as plantain doesn't require much feeding. A light application of a balanced organic fertilizer in spring is sufficient.
- **Pruning and Maintenance:** Snip off dead flowers to encourage more leaf growth. Regularly remove wilted leaves to keep the plant healthy.
- **Pest and Disease Management:** Plantain is resilient but watch for slugs and snails. Use natural repellents or barriers to protect the plants. Diseases are rare but treat any fungal infections with a fungicide.
- **Overwintering:** Plantain is perennial and will die back in winter, re-emerging in spring. No special care is needed during winter months.
- **Propagation:** Easily propagated by seed or by dividing the roots in the early spring or fall.
- **Harvesting:** Leaves can be harvested anytime during the growing season. Pick leaves before the plant flowers for best flavor and medicinal properties. Roots can be collected in autumn.
- **Climate Considerations:** Plantain is versatile and can grow in a range of climates, from cool temperate to warm regions. It adapts well to various environmental conditions and thrives in many climate zones.

How to Use Plantain

Herbal Teas or Infusions: Plantain leaves are soaked in hot water to create a healing tea that can soothe the digestive tract and respiratory issues.

Tinctures: The leaves and seeds of plantain are used to make a tincture that helps with skin irritations and promotes wound healing.

Salves-Topical Applications: Plantain leaves are infused into oils to create salves or ointments, effective for treating insect bites, stings, and cuts.

Poultices: Crushed fresh plantain leaves are applied directly to the skin to soothe and heal minor burns, wounds, and eczema.

Decoctions: A strong decoction of plantain leaves can be used as a rinse or wash for treating skin problems or as a gargle for sore throats.

Powders: Dried and powdered plantain leaves are used for their antiseptic and healing properties in herbal powders, often applied to wounds or used in dental care.

Culinary Uses: Young plantain leaves can be eaten raw in salads or cooked as a spinach alternative, providing nutritional benefits.

Ease to Grow: 1-3, Low Maintenance

Plantain is extremely easy to grow, thriving even in poor soil and requiring minimal care. It's resilient, adaptable to various climates, and can often be found growing wild in many regions. Its robust nature makes it an ideal plant for beginner gardeners or those looking for a low-maintenance herb.

Purslane

Scientifically known as Portulaca Oleracea, is a succulent, leafy plant often regarded as a weed but also valued for its nutritional and medicinal properties. It is characterized by its small, yellow flowers and fleshy, green leaves, thriving in various climates and soil types. Historically, purslane has been used in traditional medicine across many cultures, and it is notable for its high content of omega-3 fatty acids, vitamins, and minerals. This plant is often consumed in salads, soups, and stews, and has been studied for its potential health benefits, including anti-inflammatory and antioxidant effects.

Digestive System

Stomach: Purslane can aid in digestion and alleviate gastric issues due to its mucilaginous content, which soothes the stomach lining and reduces irritation.

Cardiovascular System

Blood vessels: The omega-3 fatty acids in purslane help to improve heart health by reducing blood pressure and cholesterol levels, thus benefiting the blood vessels.

Immune System

General Immunity: Purslane contains high levels of vitamin C and antioxidants, which boost the immune system's function and protect the body against infections.

How to Grow Purslane

- **Selecting the Right Variety:** Purslane (Portulaca Oleracea) comes in several varieties, with some being more suitable for culinary use due to larger leaves and a milder flavor. Golden Purslane is a popular variety for its taste and nutritional value. Starting from seeds is generally preferred as it's easy and cost-effective. Purslane seeds can be purchased from online garden retailers or local nurseries. This plant readily self-seeds and grows quickly, making it a simple choice for beginners.

- **Best Time to Plant Outdoors:** The ideal time to plant purslane outdoors is in the late spring after the last frost, when the soil has warmed up. This timing helps ensure that the young plants won't be exposed to cold temperatures that can inhibit growth.

- **Spacing Outdoor Plants:** Space purslane plants or seeds about 10 to 15 inches apart. This spacing allows each plant enough room to grow and spread out, maximizing sunlight exposure and air circulation.

- **Container Use and Soil:** Purslane thrives in well-draining soil and can do well in containers. Use a potting mix designed for succulents or make your own by mixing standard potting soil with sand to improve drainage. For outdoor gardens, amend the soil with compost to enhance fertility.

- **Sunlight and Location:** Purslane needs full sun, at least six hours of direct sunlight per day, to develop properly. It can also grow under artificial light; use a full-spectrum grow light for about 12-14 hours a day to mimic natural sunlight conditions.

- **Watering:** Water purslane moderately; it's drought-tolerant and prefers the soil to dry out between watering. Overwatering can lead to root rot, so ensure good drainage in the soil.
- **Feeding:** Fertilize purslane lightly; it doesn't require much. A balanced, all-purpose liquid fertilizer diluted to half strength can be applied monthly during the growing season.
- **Pruning and Maintenance:** Snip off dead flowers to encourage more growth and prevent the plant from self-seeding excessively. Regular pruning helps maintain a compact, bushy shape and promotes continuous leaf production.
- **Pest and Disease Management:** Purslane is relatively resistant to pests and diseases. However, watch out for common issues like aphids and leaf spot. Manage pests with insecticidal soap and treat fungal diseases by removing affected parts and improving air circulation.
- **Overwintering:** In colder climates, purslane can be grown as an annual or brought indoors to overwinter. If grown in containers, move the plant inside to a sunny spot before the first frost.
- **Propagation:** Propagate purslane through cuttings or seeds. Cuttings root easily in soil or water, making them an excellent way to expand your garden or share with friends.
- **Harvesting:** Harvest purslane leaves, stems, and flowers in the morning when their moisture content is highest. These parts are edible and rich in omega-3 fatty acids and vitamins. You can start harvesting leaves as soon as the plant reaches a suitable size, usually within a few weeks of planting.
- **Climate Considerations:** Purslane is highly adaptable and grows best in warm, sunny environments. It can tolerate heat and is less suited to cold, damp climates. Ensure the growing area receives plenty of sunlight and has good air circulation to

prevent moisture-related issues.

How to Use Purslane

Herbal Teas or Infusions: Purslane leaves and stems can be soaked in hot water to create an herbal tea. The soaking process extracts the nutrients, and the resulting tea is consumed for its health benefits.

Salves-Topical Applications: The juice from purslane leaves and stems can be used to make creams or ointments. These are applied to the skin to soothe irritations and heal wounds.

Compresses: Crushed purslane leaves can be applied directly to the skin as a compress to reduce inflammation and treat skin conditions.

Juices: Purslane can be juiced and consumed as a health drink. The juice is rich in vitamins and omega-3 fatty acids, beneficial for overall health.

Culinary Uses: Purslane is edible and can be used in salads, soups, and stews. Its leaves and stems add a slightly sour and salty flavor to dishes.

Ease to Grow: 2-3, Low Maintenance

Purslane is very easy to grow, requiring minimal care. It thrives in poor, well-drained soil and can tolerate drought conditions. Being a hardy plant, it often grows in full sun but can also tolerate partial shade, making it suitable for a variety of garden settings.

Raspberry Leaf

From the plant Rubus Idaeus, is renowned for its nutritional value and therapeutic properties. Traditionally, it has been used to support women's health, particularly during pregnancy, to ease childbirth. Its leaves are rich in vitamins, minerals, and antioxidants, making them beneficial for overall well-being. Raspberry leaf can strengthen the uterus, improve labor outcomes, and decrease childbirth complications. It's also used for its anti-inflammatory and antioxidant properties, aiding digestion and cardiovascular health. Beyond women's health, it helps in soothing sore throats, enhancing immune function, and maintaining healthy skin.

Reproductive System

Uterus: Raspberry leaf strengthens uterine muscles, facilitating labor and reducing childbirth complications.

Menstrual Health: It alleviates menstrual cramps and regulates the menstrual cycle, providing relief from PMS symptoms.

Digestive System

Gastrointestinal Tract: It soothes the digestive tract, reducing inflammation and aiding in the treatment of diarrhea and gastrointestinal disorders.

How to Grow Raspberry Leaf

- **Selecting the Right Variety:** Choose Rubus Idaeus for medicinal use; available as bare-root plants or seeds. Both methods are viable, with plants establishing faster. Purchase from reputable nurseries or online stores.
- **Best Time to Plant Outdoors:** Spring or autumn is ideal, allowing roots to establish before extreme temperatures.
- **Spacing Outdoor Plants:** Plant raspberry canes 18 inches apart in rows 6 feet apart to allow room for growth and airflow.
- **Container Use and Soil:** Use large pots with well-draining soil; mix in compost for nutrient-rich, moist conditions.
- **Sunlight and Location:** Requires full sun, at least 6-8 hours daily. Can tolerate partial shade. For artificial lighting, use full-spectrum grow lights mimicking natural sunlight.
- **Watering:** Keep soil consistently moist but not waterlogged. Water deeply once a week, more during dry spells.
- **Feeding:** Apply a balanced fertilizer in early spring and again in midsummer to support growth and fruit production.
- **Pruning and Maintenance:** Snip off dead flowers to encourage fruiting. Prune canes that have fruited once, leaving new growth for next year.
- **Pest and Disease Management:** Watch for signs like wilted leaves or spots. Treat with appropriate organic pesticides and practice good hygiene to prevent disease spread.
- **Overwintering:** In colder climates, mulch around the base to protect roots from freezing.
- **Propagation:** Propagate by division or cuttings in late winter or early spring before new growth begins.

- **Harvesting:** Leaves are best picked in late spring before blooming for maximum potency. Dry leaves for tea or use fresh.
- **Climate Considerations:** Thrives in temperate climates with cold winters and mild summers. Adapts well to different conditions but may flower too early in very warm, tropical climates.

How to Use Raspberry Leaf

Herbal Teas or Infusions: Raspberry leaf is commonly soaked in hot water to make an herbal tea known for supporting reproductive health and easing menstrual discomfort.

Tinctures: The leaves are also used to make tinctures, which are concentrated liquid extracts, taken in small doses to promote general health.

Salves-Topical Applications: Can be used in creams or ointments for skin irritation, as the leaves have anti-inflammatory properties.

Decoctions: A strong decoction of raspberry leaf can be used as a gargle or mouthwash to soothe mouth and throat inflammations.

Culinary Uses: Young tender leaves of raspberry can be added to salads or used as a culinary herb.

Ease to Grow: 2-3, Low Maintenance

Raspberry plants are quite hardy and easy to grow, requiring minimal maintenance once established. They thrive in temperate climates and can be propagated from cuttings or seeds. With basic care, raspberry plants will produce leaves that can be harvested for their medicinal properties.

Red Clover

(Trifolium Pratense) is a perennial herb renowned for its vibrant purple flowers and medicinal properties. This plant has been used traditionally in herbal medicine for various health conditions. Rich in isoflavones, vitamins, and minerals, it offers a range of health benefits.

Reproductive System

Hormonal Balance: Red Clover contains phytoestrogens that mimic estrogen, helping to balance hormonal levels and alleviate menopausal symptoms.

Cardiovascular System

Blood Flow: Its blood-thinning properties can improve circulation and help prevent blood clots.

Cholesterol: Red Clover is known to aid in reducing bad cholesterol levels, thus supporting heart health.

Respiratory System

Congestion: Acts as an expectorant, helping to clear mucus from the respiratory tract and ease breathing.

Endocrine System

Thyroid Health: It indirectly supports thyroid function due to its isoflavonoid content, which can influence hormone levels.

Skin and Integumentary System

Skin Health: Applied topically or used in baths, it can help treat skin conditions like eczema and psoriasis due to its anti-inflammatory and soothing properties.

How to Grow Red Clover

- **Selecting the Right Variety:** Red Clover (Trifolium pratense) is the most common variety used for medicinal purposes. Starting with seeds is generally preferred as it grows readily. Seeds are available online or at garden centers.
- **Best Time to Plant Outdoors:** Plant in early spring or fall when the temperature is cooler to allow the plant to establish without the stress of heat.
- **Spacing Outdoor Plants:** Space plants or seeds about 6 to 8 inches apart to allow enough room for growth and air circulation.
- **Container Use and Soil:** Red Clover thrives in well-drained soil with good fertility levels. For container gardening, use a pot with drainage holes and a standard potting mix.
- **Sunlight and Location:** Prefers full sun to partial shade, requiring at least 4-6 hours of sunlight daily. If using artificial lighting, fluorescent or LED grow lights are suitable.
- **Watering:** Keep the soil consistently moist but not waterlogged. Watering should be more frequent during dry spells.

- **Feeding:** Apply a balanced fertilizer in the spring to support growth but avoid over-fertilizing, which can lead to excessive foliage at the expense of flowers.
- **Pruning and Maintenance:** Snip off dead flowers to promote new growth and prevent the plant from flowering too early.
- **Pest and Disease Management:** Monitor for common pests like aphids and for diseases like powdery mildew. Use organic pest control methods and ensure good air circulation to prevent disease.
- **Overwintering:** In colder climates, red clover is treated as an annual, but in warmer areas, it may survive winter and regrow in spring.
- **Propagation:** Can be propagated by seed or division in spring. Seed propagation is straightforward; simply scatter seeds on prepared soil.
- **Harvesting:** Harvest flowers when they are in full bloom, typically in late spring or early summer. The flowers are used for teas, tinctures, and extracts, and are harvested for their medicinal properties, particularly for supporting women's health and aiding in respiratory issues.
- **Climate Considerations:** Thrives in temperate climates with regular rainfall, and can tolerate a range of climate conditions but prefers areas with distinct seasons and no extreme heat or cold.

How to Use Red Clover

Herbal Teas or Infusions: Red Clover flowers are soaked in hot water for several minutes to make a tea that supports respiratory and women's health.

Tinctures: The flowers are steeped in alcohol to extract their beneficial compounds, creating a potent liquid used for various health concerns.

Salves-Topical Applications: Dried flowers are infused into oils to make creams or ointments for skin conditions like eczema or psoriasis.

Decoctions: Plant parts can be boiled in water for a long time to make a strong liquid used to alleviate respiratory issues.

Syrups: A sweetened liquid prepared from the decoction is often used for soothing throat irritations and coughs.

Gargles & Mouthwashes: A solution made from the leaves or flowers is used to treat mouth ulcers and sore throats.

Ease to Grow: 2-3, Low Maintenance

Red Clover is a hardy plant that grows easily in most temperate climates. It requires minimal care once established and can thrive in a variety of soil types, making it a low-maintenance choice for both novice and experienced gardeners. Its ability to fix nitrogen also improves soil health.

Rhodiola Rosea

Commonly known as golden root or Arctic root, is a perennial flowering plant that grows in the cold, mountainous regions of Europe and Asia. It is well-regarded in traditional medicine systems for its "adaptogenic" properties, which means it helps the body resist physical, chemical, and environmental stress. The roots contain over 140 active ingredients, with salidroside and rosavin being the most prominent. Rhodiola is often used to enhance physical endurance, mental performance, and resistance to high-altitude sickness.

Nervous System

Brain Function: Rhodiola Rosea enhances cognitive functions like memory, attention, and concentration by improving neurotransmitter activity.

Endocrine System

Adrenal Glands: Supports adrenal gland function, helping the body to manage stress more effectively by regulating stress hormones.

How to Grow Rhodiola Rosea

- **Selecting the Right Variety:** Rhodiola Rosea is the most studied species, known for its adaptogenic properties. It's preferable to start with seeds or root cuttings. Purchase from reputable nurseries or online stores specializing in medicinal herbs.
- **Best Time to Plant Outdoors:** Plant in early spring after the last frost. Rhodiola requires a cold period to germinate, making spring the ideal season for planting.
- **Spacing Outdoor Plants:** Space plants or seeds about 12 inches apart to allow room for growth and adequate air circulation.
- **Container Use and Soil:** Rhodiola thrives in well-drained soil with a neutral to slightly acidic pH. In containers, use a mix of potting soil, sand, and peat to mimic its native gritty, rocky soil.

- **Sunlight and Location:** Prefers full sun to partial shade, requiring at least 6 hours of sunlight daily. In regions with intense sun, partial shade can prevent overheating.
- **Watering:** Water regularly to keep the soil moist but not waterlogged. Rhodiola is drought-tolerant once established but benefits from consistent moisture during the growing season.
- **Feeding:** Fertilize lightly in the spring with a balanced, slow-release fertilizer to support growth without overstimulating.
- **Pruning and Maintenance:** Snip off dead flowers to encourage more robust growth. Remove any dead or damaged leaves to maintain plant health.
- **Pest and Disease Management:** Watch for root rot in overly wet conditions. Ensure good drainage and airflow around the plant to prevent fungal diseases.
- **Overwintering:** In colder climates, mulch around the base to protect roots from freezing temperatures.
- **Propagation:** Propagate by dividing the roots or from seed. Root division is best done in the fall or early spring.
- **Harvesting:** The roots are the most commonly used part, harvested in the fall of the second or third year. They contain the plant's active compounds and can be dried for later use.
- **Climate Considerations:** Thrives in cold, alpine climates similar to its native Siberian habitat. Can withstand frost and prefers cool summer temperatures.

How to Use Rhodiola Rosea

Tinctures: Rhodiola rosea is commonly used in tincture form. The root is soaked in alcohol to extract the active compounds, which are then taken in small doses to help combat fatigue and stress.

Decoctions: The dried roots can be boiled in water to make a decoction. This liquid is then consumed for its adaptogenic benefits, helping the body adapt to and resist physical, chemical, and environmental stress.

Powders: Rhodiola root can be dried and ground into a powder, which is then used in capsules or mixed with water or juice. This form is taken to enhance mental performance and physical endurance.

Ease to Grow: 3-5, Medium Maintenance

Growing Rhodiola Rosea can be moderately challenging due to its preference for cold climates and specific soil conditions. It requires well-drained soil and cool temperatures, mimicking its natural alpine habitat. With proper care, it can be a rewarding herb to cultivate for its numerous health benefits.

Rosehip

Derived from the fruit of the rose plant, it is rich in vitamins, especially vitamin C, and antioxidants. It has been traditionally used in herbal medicine for its various health benefits. Rosehip is known to benefit several physiological systems:

Immune System

Immune Response: Rosehip is known for its high vitamin C content, which supports a healthy immune system and helps the body fight off infections.

Antioxidant Activity: Its antioxidants help protect cells from oxidative stress, contributing to overall immune system health.

Skin and Integumentary System

Skin Health: Rosehip oil is used topically for its moisturizing and anti-aging properties, promoting healthy skin and reducing signs of aging.

Digestive System

Digestion: Can relieve symptoms of indigestion and gastrointestinal discomfort.

Muscular System

Rosehip's anti-inflammatory properties can help reduce muscle pain and improve flexibility.

How to Grow Rosehip

- **Selecting the Right Variety:** There are many varieties of rosehip-producing plants; Rosa rugosa and Rosa Canina are popular for their large, vitamin-rich hips. Starting with nursery-grown plants is often easier than growing from seeds, as seeds require stratification (subjecting seeds to cold, moist conditions for a specific period of time before planting them) so can take a long time to germinate. Plants can be purchased from nurseries or online garden shops.
- **Best Time to Plant Outdoors:** Plant Rosehips in early spring or late autumn. This timing gives the plants a chance to establish roots before the extreme temperatures of summer or winter.

- **Spacing Outdoor Plants:** Space plants about 4 to 6 feet apart to ensure they have room to grow and receive adequate airflow, which helps prevent disease.
- **Container Use and Soil:** Rosehips can grow in containers but prefer open ground. They need well-draining soil with organic matter. Amend heavy clay or sandy soil with compost to improve fertility and drainage.
- **Sunlight and Location:** Rosehip plants require full sun, at least 6 to 8 hours of direct sunlight daily. If using artificial lighting, high-output grow lights that mimic full-spectrum sunlight are needed.
- **Watering:** Water regularly to keep the soil moist but not waterlogged, especially during dry periods. Young plants need more frequent watering until established.
- **Feeding:** Feed rosehip plants in spring with a balanced fertilizer to support growth and fruit production. Avoid over-fertilizing, which can lead to more foliage and fewer hips.
- **Pruning and Maintenance:** Prune in late winter or early spring to remove dead or weak branches and encourage new growth. Snip off dead flowers to promote healthier plants.
- **Pest and Disease Management:** Watch for rust, black spot, and aphids. Treat with appropriate fungicides or insecticides and improve air circulation to prevent these issues.
- **Overwintering:** In colder regions, mulch around the base to protect roots from freezing. Container plants may need to be moved indoors or to a protected area.
- **Propagation:** Propagate by seed in autumn or by softwood cuttings in late spring. Seeds require cold stratification before planting.
- **Harvesting:** Rosehips are harvested in late summer or fall after they have colored and softened. They are used for their seeds and flesh, which are high in vitamin C and antioxidants.

- **Climate Considerations:** Rosehips prefer a temperate climate with well-defined seasons, including cold winters and warm summers, to stimulate dormancy and fruiting.

How to Use Rosehip

Herbal Teas or Infusions: Rosehip can be soaked in hot water to create an herbal tea rich in vitamin C and antioxidants, beneficial for boosting the immune system.

Tinctures: Rosehips are also used in tinctures to extract their nutrients, offering a concentrated form for health benefits like anti-inflammation and immune support.

Salves-Topical Applications: The oil extracted from rosehip seeds is used in creams and ointments for its skin-regenerating properties, helping to improve skin elasticity and reduce scars.

Decoctions: Boiling rosehips in water makes a decoction that can be consumed for its health benefits, particularly for digestive and immune health.

Syrups: Rosehip syrup is a traditional remedy used for its high vitamin C content, aiding in cold and flu prevention and treatment.

Powders: Dried and powdered rosehip are added to food or smoothies for nutritional supplementation.

Culinary Uses: Rosehips are used in jams, jellies, and soups, providing a tangy flavor and vitamin C boost.

Ease to Grow: 3-6, Medium Maintenance

Growing rosehip plants requires some attention to ensure they thrive. They need well-draining soil, regular watering, and full sun but are relatively hardy and can withstand a range of environmental conditions once established.

Rosemary

A fragrant evergreen herb native to the Mediterranean region. Known for its needle-like leaves and woody aroma, rosemary is not only a popular culinary herb but also has a long history of use in traditional medicine. Rich in antioxidants and anti-inflammatory compounds, it's believed to boost the immune system, improve digestion, and enhance memory and concentration. Its essential oil is used for its aromatic and therapeutic properties.

Digestive System

Stomach: Rosemary stimulates digestion, helps to relieve bloating and flatulence, and can calm an upset stomach.

Nervous System

Brain: Enhances memory and concentration by increasing blood flow to the brain, and has antioxidant properties that may protect neural cells.

Respiratory System

Lungs: Acts as an expectorant, helping to clear mucus and relieve congestion in the respiratory tract.

Skin and Integumentary System

Skin: Its antibacterial and anti-inflammatory properties help to heal skin conditions, and its antioxidant content aids in reducing skin aging.

How to Grow Rosemary

- **Selecting the Right Variety:** There are several varieties of rosemary, including 'Tuscan Blue', 'Miss Jessopp's Upright', and 'Prostratus', each with unique growth habits and flavors. Starting from cuttings or purchasing young plants from nurseries or garden centers is generally more successful than growing from seeds.

- **Best Time to Plant Outdoors:** Plant rosemary in spring or early summer to allow it to establish before cold weather. In warmer climates, it can also be planted in the fall.

- **Spacing Outdoor Plants:** Space rosemary plants 2 to 3 feet apart to ensure adequate air circulation and room for growth.

- **Container Use and Soil:** Rosemary thrives in well-draining soil and can be grown in containers. Use a potting mix designed for herbs or succulents. Ensure pots have drainage holes.

- **Sunlight and Location:** Rosemary requires full sun, at least 6-8 hours daily. If using artificial lighting, LED or fluorescent grow lights are effective, mimicking natural sunlight.

- **Watering:** Water rosemary plants deeply but infrequently, allowing the soil to dry out between watering. Overwatering can lead to root rot.

- **Feeding:** Rosemary does not require frequent fertilization. A light application of a balanced, slow-release fertilizer in the spring can support growth.

- **Pruning and Maintenance:** Regular pruning helps maintain shape and promotes dense growth. Snip off dead flowers to encourage new growth and prevent the plant from flowering too early.
- **Pest and Disease Management:** Rosemary is generally resistant to pests and diseases. However, watch for aphids and spider mites. Use insecticidal soap or neem oil for treatment.
- **Overwintering:** In colder climates, protect rosemary in winter by mulching or bringing containers indoors. Ensure the plant is in a cool, well-ventilated area with plenty of light.
- **Propagation:** Propagate rosemary from cuttings in late spring or early summer. Remove the lower leaves and place cuttings in a well-draining soil mix.
- **Harvesting:** Harvest rosemary sprigs as needed. The best time to collect large quantities is just before the plant flowers when the oils are most concentrated in the leaves.
- **Climate Considerations:** Rosemary prefers a warm, sunny climate but can tolerate cold with proper winter protection. It thrives in temperatures ranging from 55 to 80 degrees Fahrenheit.

How to Use Rosemary

Herbal Teas or Infusions: Soak rosemary leaves in boiling water to create a tea that can help improve digestion and enhance memory and concentration.

Tinctures: Rosemary leaves are soaked in alcohol to extract their active compounds, creating a concentrated tincture that can be used for its antioxidant and anti-inflammatory properties.

Salves-Topical Applications: Infused in oils, rosemary can be made into salves or creams for topical application to alleviate muscle pain, improve circulation, and provide antiseptic benefits.

Compresses: A cloth soaked in a rosemary infusion can be applied to areas of the skin to reduce inflammation and ease pain.

Aromatherapy & Essential Oils: Rosemary essential oil is used in diffusers or applied topically when diluted with a carrier oil to improve mental clarity, relieve stress, and stimulate hair growth.

Herbal Baths: Adding rosemary to bathwater can help relieve sore muscles, improve circulation, and provide a refreshing and rejuvenating experience.

Steam Inhalation: Inhaling steam infused with rosemary essential oil or leaves can clear nasal passages and help relieve respiratory conditions.

Decoctions: Boiling rosemary in water for a prolonged period extracts its potent compounds, creating a strong decoction used for its health benefits, particularly in digestive health.

Syrups: Rosemary can be incorporated into syrups to soothe coughs or sore throats due to its antimicrobial and anti-inflammatory properties.

Gargles & Mouthwashes: A rosemary infusion can be used as a gargle or mouthwash to improve oral health, reducing inflammation and killing bacteria.

Culinary Uses: Rosemary is widely used in cooking for its aromatic flavor, enhancing meats, soups, breads, and more.

Ease to Grow: 2-4, Low Maintenance

Rosemary is relatively easy to grow, requiring minimal maintenance. It thrives in well-drained soil, needs full sun, and prefers infrequent watering, making it a low-maintenance plant ideal for beginners. Its resilience and aromatic leaves make it a popular choice in both culinary and medicinal applications.

Saffron

Derived from the flower of Crocus sativus, is a highly prized spice known for its distinct aroma, color, and flavor. Beyond its culinary use, saffron has medicinal properties and is used in traditional medicine to treat various ailments. Its bioactive compounds, including crocin, crocetin, and safranal, contribute to its health benefits.

Nervous System
Brain: Saffron is known to enhance mood, alleviate depression, and improve memory and cognitive function by affecting neurotransmitters and protecting against oxidative stress.

Digestive System
Stomach: It can help alleviate gastric issues and improve digestion by reducing inflammation and acting as an antispasmodic agent.

Cardiovascular System
Blood Vessels: Saffron helps regulate cholesterol levels and blood pressure, improving circulation and reducing the risk of heart diseases.

Reproductive System
Reproductive Organs: In traditional medicine, saffron is used to alleviate menstrual discomfort and regulate periods.

How to Grow Saffron

- **Selecting the Right Variety:** Saffron is obtained from the Crocus Sativus plant. There are not many varieties to choose from, and the main focus should be on obtaining high-quality corms, which are the bulb-like structures of the plant. It's preferable to start with corms rather than seeds as it ensures the plant will produce saffron threads. These can be purchased from reputable nurseries or online stores specializing in herbs and spices.

- **Best Time to Plant Outdoors:** The best time to plant saffron corms is in late summer or early fall. This timing allows the plant to establish itself and flower in the fall.

- **Spacing Outdoor Plants:** Plant the corms about 4 inches deep and 6 inches apart in well-drained soil to prevent rot.

- **Container Use and Soil:** Saffron can be grown in containers if outdoor space is limited. Use well-draining potting soil and ensure the container has adequate drainage holes. The soil should be rich in organic matter.

- **Sunlight and Location:** Saffron requires full sunlight, needing at least 6 hours of direct sunlight each day. If growing indoors, use grow lights to supplement sunlight.

- **Watering:** Water the corms sparingly to keep the soil slightly moist but not waterlogged, as saffron does not tolerate wet roots.

- **Feeding:** Apply a balanced, slow-release fertilizer at the beginning of the growing season to support growth.

- **Pruning and Maintenance:** Snip off dead flowers to promote more flowering. Remove any dead or diseased plant material to keep the plant healthy.

- **Pest and Disease Management:** Watch for signs of rot or mildew, which can appear as moldy patches or soft, brown areas on the corms and plants. Ensure good air circulation and avoid overwatering to prevent these issues.

- **Overwintering:** In colder climates, mulch around the plants to protect the corms from freezing temperatures.
- **Propagation:** Propagate saffron by dividing and replanting the corms every three to four years to prevent overcrowding and to rejuvenate the planting.
- **Harvesting:** Harvest the saffron stigmas (threads) in the morning when the flowers are open. Use tweezers to gently pluck the red stigmas from the center of each flower. Dry them for use as a spice or for medicinal purposes.
- **Climate Considerations:** Saffron grows best in climates with hot, dry summers and cool to cold winters. It does not thrive in tropical or overly humid conditions.

How to Use Saffron

Herbal Teas or Infusions: Saffron can be soaked in hot water to make a golden-hued tea. This infusion is often consumed for its potential mood-enhancing and antioxidant properties.

Culinary Uses: Saffron is extensively used in cooking for its unique flavor and color. It's a staple in dishes like paella, risotto, and various Middle Eastern and South Asian cuisines.

Ease to Grow: 6-8, Medium to High Maintenance

Growing saffron requires specific climatic conditions and careful attention. It thrives in regions with a pronounced seasonal change, needing hot, dry summers and cool winters. The cultivation process is labor-intensive, primarily due to the manual harvesting of the stigmas, which are the parts of the plant used to produce saffron.

Sage

Known scientifically as Salvia Officinalis, is a perennial herb with a long history of culinary and medicinal use. It is characterized by its woody stems, grayish leaves, and a strong, earthy fragrance. Traditionally, sage has been used to improve memory, aid digestion, and treat inflammation. Its antimicrobial properties make it beneficial in treating throat infections and dental abscesses.

Digestive System

Stomach: Sage stimulates digestion, relieves indigestion, and reduces gas and bloating.

Liver: Aids the liver by promoting detoxification, reducing inflammation, supporting digestion, and providing antioxidant protection against oxidative stress.

Nervous System

Brain: Sage has been shown to improve memory and cognitive function, particularly in individuals with Alzheimer's disease.

Respiratory System

Throat: Sage acts as an anti-inflammatory and antimicrobial agent, helping to soothe sore throats and treat oral infections.

Immune System

General Immune Support: Sage contains compounds that boost the immune system and protect against microbial infections.

Skin and Integumentary System

Skin: Sage's antimicrobial and anti-inflammatory properties aid in the healing of skin wounds and infections.

How to Grow Sage

- **Selecting the Right Variety:** Common varieties of sage include garden sage, purple sage, and golden sage. Garden sage is most widely used for culinary purposes. Seeds or starter plants can be purchased from nurseries or online garden stores.
- **Best Time to Plant Outdoors:** Plant sage in spring after the last frost, or in early fall in warmer climates.
- **Spacing Outdoor Plants:** Space sage plants 18 to 24 inches apart to allow for proper air circulation and growth.
- **Container Use and Soil:** Sage thrives in well-draining soil with a pH between 6.0 and 7.0. It can be grown in containers using a potting mix designed for herbs.
- **Sunlight and Location:** Sage requires full sun, at least 6 to 8 hours of direct sunlight daily. If using artificial lighting, LED grow lights are effective.
- **Watering:** Allow the soil to dry out between waterings. Sage prefers drier conditions and is drought-tolerant.
- **Feeding:** Apply a balanced, slow-release fertilizer at the beginning of the growing season to support growth.
- **Pruning and Maintenance:** Regularly snip off dead flowers to encourage new growth and prevent the plant from flowering too early.

- **Pest and Disease Management:** Watch for common issues like powdery mildew and spider mites. Treat with appropriate organic pesticides or fungicides as needed.
- **Overwintering:** In colder zones, mulch around the base to protect roots in winter. Potted plants can be moved indoors.
- **Propagation:** Sage can be propagated from cuttings or by division in early spring.
- **Harvesting:** Leaves can be harvested as needed. Pick leaves in the morning for the best flavor and aroma. Leaves, stems, and flowers are all usable.
- **Climate Considerations:** Sage grows best in climates with warm, sunny days and cool nights. It does not thrive in extremely humid or very wet conditions.

How to Use Sage

Herbal Teas or Infusions: Soak dried or fresh sage leaves in boiling water for 5-10 minutes to make a soothing tea that can aid digestion and relieve sore throats.

Tinctures: Sage leaves are soaked in alcohol to extract the active compounds, creating a tincture that can be used for its antimicrobial and anti-inflammatory properties.

Salves-Topical Applications: Infused in oils, sage can be made into salves or ointments to treat skin conditions like eczema or acne due to its anti-inflammatory properties.

Compresses: A cloth soaked in sage-infused water can be applied to areas of inflammation or wounds to reduce swelling and promote healing.

Decoctions: Boiling sage leaves in water makes a strong decoction that can be used as a rinse for gingivitis or throat infections.

Gargles & Mouthwashes: A sage infusion can be used as a gargle or mouthwash to alleviate sore throats, reduce dental plaque, and treat mouth ulcers.

Culinary Uses: Sage is commonly used in cooking for its aromatic flavor, especially in dishes like stuffing, sauces, and poultry seasoning.

Ease to Grow: 2-4, Low Maintenance

Sage is a hardy plant that thrives in well-draining soil and full sunlight. It requires minimal watering once established and is relatively low maintenance, making it an excellent choice for beginner gardeners. Sage's aromatic leaves can be harvested for culinary and medicinal uses.

Schisandra

Also known as Schisandra Chinensis, is a plant native to East Asia, renowned for its adaptogenic properties that help the body resist stressors of various kinds, including physical, chemical, and biological. The berries of the Schisandra plant are used for their health benefits, as they contain lignans and other compounds that are beneficial for human health. They are often used in traditional Chinese medicine to enhance energy, improve vision, and stimulate the immune system. Schisandra berries are known for their distinctive five-flavor taste, which includes sweet, salty, sour, pungent, and bitter.

Nervous System

Brain: Schisandra enhances mental performance, improving concentration, memory, and alertness by stimulating the central nervous system.

Endocrine System

Adrenal Glands: Schisandra has adaptogenic effects (adapt to stress and maintain overall mental well-being), helping to balance hormones and improve the body's response to stress.

Immune System

General Immunity: The antioxidants in Schisandra enhance the immune system by fighting free radicals and reducing inflammation.

How to Grow Schisandra

- **Selecting the Right Variety:** Schisandra Chinensis is the commonly cultivated variety known for its medicinal properties. Preferable to start with seeds, although starts are also an option. Seeds and plants can be purchased from specialty nurseries or online retailers.
- **Best Time to Plant Outdoors:** Plant in late winter or early spring after the last frost. This timing allows the plant to establish before summer.
- **Spacing Outdoor Plants:** Space plants 3 to 6 feet apart to allow room for growth and airflow, reducing the risk of disease.
- **Container Use and Soil:** Schisandra grows well in containers if outdoor space is limited. Use well-draining soil with a mix of peat, sand, and compost to ensure good root health.
- **Sunlight and Location:** Prefers partial shade, especially in hotter climates, with around 4-6 hours of sunlight daily. Can tolerate full sun in cooler regions.

- **Watering:** Keep the soil consistently moist but not waterlogged. Water deeply once a week, more frequently during dry spells.
- **Feeding:** Apply a balanced, slow-release fertilizer in the early spring and again in mid-summer to support growth and berry production.
- **Pruning and Maintenance:** Snip off dead flowers to promote new growth and prevent the plant from investing energy into seed production.
- **Pest and Disease Management:** Watch for common garden pests like aphids and spider mites. Treat with organic insecticidal soap or neem oil. For disease, ensure good air circulation and avoid overhead watering to prevent fungal issues.
- **Overwintering:** In colder climates, mulch heavily around the base to protect roots from freezing temperatures.
- **Propagation:** Can be propagated by seed, softwood cuttings in spring, or hardwood cuttings in late fall.
- **Harvesting:** Harvest berries in late summer when they turn bright red. Berries are the primary part used for their medicinal properties, often dried or processed into extracts or teas.
- **Climate Considerations:** Thrives in temperate climates with cold winters and prefers well-defined seasons to stimulate the dormancy and active growth cycle.

How to Use Schisandra

Herbal Teas or Infusions: Schisandra berries are soaked in hot water to create an herbal tea known for its adaptogenic properties, enhancing stress resistance and boosting energy.

Tinctures: The berries are used to make tinctures, offering a concentrated form of its benefits, particularly for liver health and stress reduction.

Decoctions: Schisandra berries are boiled in water to make a strong decoction, used traditionally to improve respiratory and liver function.

Powders: Dried Schisandra berries are ground into a fine powder, which can be added to foods or drinks for an antioxidant boost.

Culinary Uses: The berries are sometimes used in small amounts in culinary dishes for their unique flavor and health properties.

Ease to Grow: 5-7, Medium Maintenance

Growing Schisandra can be moderately challenging, requiring attention to climatic conditions, soil type, and moisture levels. It prefers a cool, temperate climate and can take several years to start producing fruit, needing support structures for its vine-like growth habit.

Shepherd's Purse

(Capsella bursa-pastoris) is a small, herbaceous plant recognized for its heart-shaped seed pouches. Thriving in various environments, it is often found in gardens, roadsides, and fields. This plant is valued in herbal medicine, primarily for its hemostatic properties, which help to stop bleeding. Shepherd's Purse contains flavonoids, glycosides, and volatile oils, contributing to its therapeutic effects.

Reproductive System

Uterus: Shepherd's Purse is known for its ability to reduce uterine bleeding and is often used to treat heavy menstrual flows.

Cardiovascular System

Blood Vessels: The herb acts as a vasoconstrictor, helping to narrow blood vessels and reduce bleeding.

How to Grow Shepherd's Purse

- **Selecting the Right Variety:** Shepherd's Purse is typically found in one common variety. It is generally grown from seeds rather than starts. Seeds are available at online herb and garden stores.
- **Best Time to Plant Outdoors:** Plant in early spring or fall. The cool temperatures help to establish the plant.
- **Spacing Outdoor Plants:** Space plants or seeds about 6 to 8 inches apart to allow enough room for growth.
- **Container Use and Soil:** Thrives in well-drained soil with a neutral pH. Containers should have good drainage holes.
- **Sunlight and Location:** Requires full sun to partial shade, with around 4 to 6 hours of sunlight daily. Can be grown under artificial grow lights if necessary.
- **Watering:** Water regularly to keep the soil moist but not waterlogged. Reduce watering once plants are established.
- **Feeding:** Fertilize lightly; too much can reduce the concentration of medicinal compounds in the plant.
- **Pruning and Maintenance:** Snip off dead flowers to encourage more growth and prevent the plant from seeding too early.

- **Pest and Disease Management:** Monitor for common pests like aphids. Treat diseases early, such as rot, by improving soil drainage or using organic fungicides.
- **Overwintering:** In colder climates, mulch around the base to protect roots from freezing temperatures.
- **Propagation:** Easily propagated by seed. Allow some plants to flower and seed to encourage self-sowing.
- **Harvesting:** Leaves can be harvested throughout the growing season; the entire plant can be used, including leaves, stems, and seeds, especially before it flowers for optimal potency.
- **Climate Considerations:** Best in temperate climates; does not require a specific zone but thrives in areas with distinct seasons.

How to Use Shepherd's Purse

Herbal Teas or Infusions: Shepherd's Purse leaves can be soaked in hot water to make tea, which is often used to help with menstrual and digestive issues.

Tinctures: The aerial parts of the plant (above ground portions) are used to make tinctures, which can support circulatory health and manage bleeding.

Salves-Topical Applications: Crushed fresh leaves or extracts are used in salves or ointments to treat wounds and bruises due to its astringent properties.

Poultices: Fresh or dried leaves can be applied directly to the skin as a poultice for cuts, scrapes, and hemorrhoids.

Decoctions: A decoction made from the plant can be used to ease nosebleeds and urinary problems.

Powders: Dried and powdered Shepherd's Purse can be used on wounds to promote healing and reduce bleeding.

Ease to Grow: 1-3, Low Maintenance

Shepherd's Purse is a hardy plant, easy to cultivate in a variety of soil conditions and climates. It requires minimal care, making it an excellent choice for beginner gardeners. It's known for its rapid growth and ability to thrive even in poor soil.

Skullcap

Scientifically known as Scutellaria, is a perennial herb with a rich history in herbal medicine, particularly within traditional Chinese and Native American practices. Recognized for its delicate blue flowers and helmet-shaped calyx, skullcap thrives in moist, rich soils across North America and parts of Europe. It's commonly used in herbalism for its sedative and anti-inflammatory properties. Skullcap has garnered attention for its potential to alleviate anxiety, insomnia, and various nervous disorders, thanks to its active compounds like scutellarin and baicalin which contribute to its therapeutic effects.

Nervous System

Brain: Skullcap may enhance mood and reduce anxiety by modulating neurotransmitter activity.

Nerves: Known for its calming effects, it may help soothe nervous tension and prevent convulsions.

How to Grow Skullcap

- **Selecting the Right Variety:** Common skullcap (Scutellaria Lateriflora) and Baikal skullcap (Scutellaria Baicalensis) are beneficial varieties. Seeds are typically used for propagation. Available for purchase online or at specialty herb nurseries.
- **Best Time to Plant Outdoors:** Plant in spring after the last frost to ensure seedling survival and optimal growth.
- **Spacing Outdoor Plants:** Space plants or seeds 12 to 18 inches apart to allow for full growth and adequate air circulation.
- **Container Use and Soil:** Prefers well-draining, loamy soil with a neutral pH. Suitable for container gardening if ample space and consistent moisture are maintained.
- **Sunlight and Location:** Thrives in full sun to partial shade, needing about 6 to 8 hours of sunlight daily. If using artificial light, LED grow lights are effective.
- **Watering:** Keep the soil consistently moist but not waterlogged. Water when the top inch of soil feels dry to the touch.
- **Feeding:** Apply a balanced, slow-release fertilizer at the beginning of the growing season to support growth.
- **Pruning and Maintenance:** Snip off dead flowers to encourage new growth and prevent the plant from flowering too early.
- **Pest and Disease Management:** Monitor for common pests like aphids and spider mites. Treat diseases like root rot by improving soil drainage and reducing watering.
- **Overwintering:** In colder climates, mulch around the base to protect roots from freezing temperatures.

- **Propagation:** Easily propagated by seed in spring or by dividing roots in fall or early spring.
- **Harvesting:** Leaves and flowers can be harvested in summer when the plant is in bloom. Use them fresh or dried for their medicinal properties.
- **Climate Considerations:** Best grown in temperate climates with distinct seasons. Does not thrive in extremely hot or tropical environments.

How to Use Skullcap

Herbal Teas or Infusions: Leaves are soaked in hot water to create a calming tea, commonly used to reduce anxiety and promote sleep.

Tinctures: The aerial parts of skullcap are extracted into alcohol to create a tincture, used for its sedative and anti-inflammatory properties.

Salves-Topical Applications: Infused oils from skullcap can be used in salves or ointments to soothe skin irritations and inflammation.

Decoctions: A strong tea made by boiling the plant's leaves or roots, used traditionally to aid digestion and relieve respiratory conditions.

Powders: Dried and ground skullcap can be used in powdered form, often encapsulated as a dietary supplement for nervous system support.

Ease to Grow: 3-5, Low Maintenance

Skullcap is a resilient plant that adapts well to various conditions but prefers a moist, well-drained environment and partial shade. It's relatively low maintenance, making it a good choice for beginner gardeners.

Slippery Elm

Also known as Ulmus Rubra, is a tree native to North America known for its dark brown to reddish-brown bark. The inner bark has been used medicinally for centuries, particularly by Native American tribes. It contains a substance called mucilage, a gel-like polysaccharide that becomes a slick gel when mixed with water. This property makes it an effective remedy for soothing mucous membranes.

Digestive System

Stomach: Slippery Elm coats and soothes the stomach lining, helping to relieve gastritis, peptic ulcers, and acid reflux.

Intestines: Acts as a gentle laxative, aids in easing constipation, and helps with the healing of hemorrhoids and irritable bowel syndrome (IBS).

Respiratory System

Throat: The mucilage in Slippery Elm soothes sore throats and alleviates coughing by coating the irritated tissues.

Lungs: It can ease the symptoms of bronchitis and asthma by soothing inflamed airways.

Skin and Integumentary System

Skin: Applied topically, it treats burns, boils, ulcers, and wounds, promoting faster healing and reducing inflammation.

How to Grow Slippery Elm

- **Selecting the Right Variety:** Slippery Elm (Ulmus Rubra) is typically the variety used for medicinal purposes. It is usually propagated through seeds rather than starts. Seeds can be purchased from reputable nurseries or online stores specializing in medicinal plants.
- **Best Time to Plant Outdoors:** Plant seeds in late fall so they can stratify (subjecting seeds to a period of cold or moist conditions to break dormancy and encourage germination) over winter and germinate in spring. In climates without freezing temperatures, plant in late winter or early spring.
- **Spacing Outdoor Plants:** Trees should be spaced at least 20 to 30 feet apart to accommodate their mature size and to ensure adequate air circulation.
- **Container Use and Soil:** Slippery Elm can be started in containers but eventually needs to be planted in the ground. Use well-draining soil, rich in organic matter. It prefers slightly acidic to neutral pH.
- **Sunlight and Location:** Requires full sun to partial shade. At least 4 to 6 hours of direct sunlight per day is ideal. If using artificial lighting, use grow lights that mimic natural sunlight.
- **Watering:** Keep the soil consistently moist, especially during the first few years of growth. Mature trees are somewhat drought tolerant but perform best with regular watering.
- **Feeding:** Apply a balanced, slow-release fertilizer in early spring to support growth. Avoid over-fertilizing which can lead to weak growth and fewer medicinal properties in the bark.

- **Pruning and Maintenance:** Prune in late winter to remove dead or crossing branches and to maintain shape. Regularly check for and remove any suckers at the base.
- **Pest and Disease Management:** Watch for signs of Dutch elm disease, characterized by yellowing leaves that wilt and fall off. Treat with appropriate fungicides and by removing affected limbs.
- **Overwintering:** Mulch around the base to protect roots in colder climates. Slippery Elm is hardy and doesn't require winter protection in most zones.
- **Propagation:** Best propagated from seed. Cuttings and grafting are less successful due to the tree's high susceptibility to disease.
- **Harvesting:** Harvest the inner bark in spring from branches or trees that are at least 10 years old. The bark is stripped and dried for medicinal use.
- **Climate Considerations:** Thrives in temperate climates with well-defined seasons. Not suitable for tropical or extreme desert climates.

How to Use Slippery Elm

Herbal Teas or Infusions: Slippery Elm bark is soaked in hot water to form a mucilaginous tea, soothing for the digestive and respiratory tracts.

Poultices: The powdered bark is mixed with water to form a paste and applied to the skin to soothe irritations and inflammations.

Decoctions: Bark is simmered in water for an extended period to extract a concentrated liquid, used to soothe sore throats and digestive issues.

Syrups: The inner bark decoction is mixed with sweeteners to make a syrup, easing cough and throat pain.

Powders: The dried bark is ground into a powder, used internally for digestive health or externally as a healing dust for wounds.

Ease to Grow: 4-6, Medium Maintenance

Growing Slippery Elm is moderately easy, requiring attention to water, soil, and spacing. It is adaptable but needs management against pests and diseases to thrive.

Soapwort

Known as Saponaria Officinalis, is a perennial herb found in Europe and Asia. With its attractive pink or white flowers, it has been traditionally used in medicine and as a natural soap due to its saponin content. Historically, soapwort was employed for washing clothes and treating skin conditions like eczema and acne because of its gentle cleansing properties. In herbal medicine, soapwort's roots and leaves have been utilized to treat various ailments, demonstrating its versatility and beneficial qualities.

Skin and Integumentary System

Skin: Soapwort contains saponins, which have cleansing and anti-inflammatory properties, helping to soothe skin irritations and conditions like eczema and acne.

How to Grow Soapwort

- **Selecting the Right Variety:** Soapwort (Saponaria Officinalis) is the most common variety used for both ornamental and medicinal purposes. It's preferable to start with seeds or plant divisions. Seeds and plants are available online or at garden centers.
- **Best Time to Plant Outdoors:** Plant soapwort seeds or starts in the spring or early fall when the soil is cool.
- **Spacing Outdoor Plants:** Space plants or seeds about 12 to 24 inches apart to allow room for growth.
- **Container Use and Soil:** Soapwort thrives in well-drained, loamy soil. It can be grown in containers using standard potting mix. Ensure pots have good drainage holes.
- **Sunlight and Location:** Prefers full sun to partial shade. In very hot climates, afternoon shade is beneficial. If using artificial lighting, LED grow lights can provide adequate light for growth.
- **Watering:** Water regularly to keep the soil moist but not waterlogged. Reduce watering in winter when the plant is dormant.
- **Feeding:** Apply a balanced liquid fertilizer monthly during the growing season.
- **Pruning and Maintenance:** Snip off dead flowers to encourage new blooms and prevent self-seeding.
- **Pest and Disease Management:** Monitor for common garden pests and fungal diseases. Soapwort is relatively pest-resistant but watch for signs of powdery mildew or leaf spot and treat with fungicides if necessary.
- **Overwintering:** In colder climates, mulch around the base to protect roots from freezing.

- **Propagation:** Easily propagated by seed or division in spring or autumn.
- **Harvesting:** Harvest leaves and flowers in the blooming season, usually in late spring or early summer. The roots can be harvested in autumn. The plant parts are used for their medicinal properties and as a natural soap.
- **Climate Considerations:** Soapwort is hardy and adaptable but thrives in temperate climates. It can withstand cold winters and hot summers but performs best with mild conditions.

How to Use Soapwort

Herbal Teas or Infusions: Soapwort leaves and flowers can be soaked in hot water for 10 minutes to make a mild tea, often used for its gentle cleansing properties.

Tinctures: A tincture can be made from the leaves and roots, typically used for skin conditions due to its soothing effects.

Salves-Topical Applications: The plant's extract is used in creams or ointments for skin irritations and rashes due to its anti-inflammatory properties.

Decoctions: Boiling the roots creates a strong decoction, historically used for cleaning purposes and sometimes for treating skin issues.

Syrups: A syrup made from soapwort extract can be used as a mild expectorant for coughs.

Culinary Uses: While not commonly consumed, soapwort's leaves have been used traditionally in small amounts to flavor soups or stews.

Ease to Grow: 2-4, Low Maintenance

Soapwort is an unassuming plant that thrives in a variety of environments, making it an excellent choice for novice gardeners. It is low maintenance, requires minimal care, and is resilient against most pests and diseases, ensuring successful cultivation with basic gardening practices.

Sorrel

(Rumex Acetosa) is a perennial herb known for its tart, lemony leaves. It's cultivated as a leafy green in many parts of the world and has a long history of culinary and medicinal uses. Sorrel is rich in vitamin C and also contains vitamins A and B, along with essential minerals like potassium and magnesium. It has been used traditionally to aid digestion, enhance the immune system, and improve skin health.

Digestive System

Stomach: Sorrel can stimulate digestion and increase appetite by promoting the secretion of gastric juices.

Immune System

General Immunity: The high vitamin C content in sorrel helps strengthen the immune system, enhancing the body's ability to fight infections.

Skin and Integumentary System

Skin: Sorrel's anti-inflammatory properties can help treat skin conditions like eczema and acne. It promotes healing and reduces inflammation.

How to Grow Sorrel

- **Selecting the Right Variety:** Sorrel comes in several varieties, with Garden Sorrel and French Sorrel being popular for their culinary use. Garden Sorrel has larger leaves, while French Sorrel is smaller and more delicate in flavor. Starting from seeds is common, but young plants or starts can also be used for quicker harvest. Seeds and plants can be purchased from garden centers or online nurseries.
- **Best Time to Plant Outdoors:** The best time to plant sorrel outdoors is in early spring, as soon as the soil can be worked. Sorrel can handle light frost and grows well in cool temperatures.
- **Spacing Outdoor Plants:** Plant sorrel seeds or starts about 12 to 18 inches apart to ensure enough space for growth and air circulation, which helps prevent disease.
- **Container Use and Soil:** Sorrel can grow in containers using standard potting soil. Ensure the soil is well-draining, as sorrel prefers moist but not waterlogged conditions. Amend with compost to increase nutrient content.
- **Sunlight and Location:** Sorrel needs full sun to partial shade, with at least 6 hours of sunlight daily. If using artificial light, provide LED grow lights for 12-14 hours per day to mimic natural sunlight.
- **Watering:** Keep the soil consistently moist but not soaked. Water sorrel plants when the top inch of soil feels dry to the touch.

- **Feeding:** Fertilize sorrel with a balanced, all-purpose liquid fertilizer once a month during the growing season to support its leaf production.
- **Pruning and Maintenance:** Regularly snip off dead flowers to encourage new growth and prevent the plant from flowering too early, which can affect the flavor of the leaves.
- **Pest and Disease Management:** Watch for common pests like aphids and treat with insecticidal soap as needed. Sorrel can be susceptible to rust; remove affected leaves and improve air circulation to manage the disease.
- **Overwintering:** In colder climates, mulch around the base of sorrel plants to protect them during winter. In very cold regions, consider growing sorrel as an annual or move containers indoors.
- **Propagation:** Sorrel can be propagated by seed, division, or root cuttings. Dividing the plants in early spring or fall can help manage their size and invigorate growth.
- **Harvesting:** Harvest sorrel leaves when they are young and tender for the best flavor. Leaves can be picked individually as needed, starting in late spring through early fall. Regular harvesting encourages new growth and can extend the productive life of the plant.
- **Climate Considerations:** Sorrel grows best in climates with distinct seasons and does well in cooler conditions. It prefers a balance of sunny and partly shaded environments, with well-drained soil and consistent moisture.

How to Use Sorrel

Herbal Teas or Infusions: Sorrel leaves can be soaked in hot water to create an herbal tea. This tea is consumed for its tangy flavor and potential health benefits, including aiding digestion and boosting vitamin C intake.

Decoctions: Sorrel leaves can be boiled in water to make a decoction, which can be used to alleviate various health issues, such as reducing inflammation and treating skin conditions.

Juices: The leaves of sorrel are juiced and consumed for their high content of vitamins and minerals, particularly beneficial for boosting energy and immune health.

Culinary Uses: Sorrel is widely used in cooking for its sharp, lemon-like flavor. It's added to soups, salads, sauces, and omelets, providing a tangy taste and a boost of nutrients.

Ease to Grow: 2-3, Low Maintenance

Sorrel is an easy-to-grow plant that adapts well to various soil types and environmental conditions. It requires minimal care, thriving in full sun to partial shade and preferring well-drained soil. Regular watering and occasional feeding will support its growth, making it a low-maintenance choice for gardeners.

Spearmint

Scientifically known as Mentha spicata, is a perennial herb with a distinct sweet flavor. Known for its aromatic leaves, spearmint is widely used in cooking, teas, and herbal remedies. It thrives in full sun to partial shade and prefers moist, well-drained soil. Spearmint's cooling menthol makes it a favorite in culinary and medicinal applications. It is easier to grow compared to other mints, spreading quickly and can become invasive if not managed. Besides its culinary use, spearmint has therapeutic benefits, including digestive and respiratory relief.

Digestive System

Stomach: Spearmint aids in relieving symptoms of indigestion, nausea, and stomachaches by relaxing the digestive tract muscles.

Respiratory System

Lungs: The menthol in spearmint acts as an expectorant, helping to clear mucus and ease breathing.

Nervous System

Brain: Spearmint has been shown to improve memory and cognitive function, possibly due to its antioxidant properties.

How to Grow Spearmint

- **Selecting the Right Variety:** Spearmint varieties include 'Native' and 'Scotch' spearmint, known for their flavor and aroma. Seeds or starts are suitable, with starts often providing quicker growth. Purchase from reputable nurseries or online stores specializing in herbs.
- **Best Time to Plant Outdoors:** Plant spearmint in the spring after the last frost to ensure a growing season long enough for the plant to establish itself.
- **Spacing Outdoor Plants:** Space plants or seeds 18 to 24 inches apart to allow room for growth and air circulation, reducing the risk of fungal diseases.

- **Container Use and Soil:** Grow in containers with well-draining potting mix to control spread. Outdoor soil should be fertile, moist, and well-draining.
- **Sunlight and Location:** Spearmint prefers full sun to partial shade, requiring at least 4-6 hours of sunlight daily. If using artificial light, provide 14-16 hours of light to mimic summer conditions.
- **Watering:** Keep the soil consistently moist but not waterlogged. Water when the top inch of soil feels dry to the touch.
- **Feeding:** Apply a balanced, water-soluble fertilizer monthly during the growing season to support vigorous growth.
- **Pruning and Maintenance:** Regularly snip off dead flowers to encourage bushier growth and prevent the plant from flowering too early.
- **Pest and Disease Management:** Watch for aphids and spider mites. Treat infestations with insecticidal soap and remove affected parts. Prevent root rot by ensuring good drainage.
- **Overwintering:** In colder climates, mulch around the base to protect roots from freezing. Container plants can be moved indoors.
- **Propagation:** Propagate by dividing established plants or rooting stem cuttings in water or soil to expand your collection.
- **Harvesting:** Harvest leaves as needed throughout the growing season. The leaves are most flavorful before the plant flowers. Use leaves fresh or dried for teas, culinary dishes, and herbal remedies.
- **Climate Considerations:** Thrives in temperate climates with consistent moisture. Avoid extreme cold or dry conditions.

How to Use Spearmint

Herbal Teas or Infusions: Spearmint leaves are soaked in hot water for several minutes to make a refreshing tea known for its digestive and relaxing properties.

Tinctures: Spearmint leaves are steeped in alcohol to extract their essential oils, creating a concentrated liquid used for its therapeutic benefits.

Salves-Topical Applications: Spearmint is infused into creams or ointments to apply on the skin, offering a cooling sensation and relief from minor irritations.

Compresses: A cloth soaked in a spearmint infusion is applied to the skin to soothe and reduce discomfort in affected areas.

Aromatherapy & Essential Oils: Spearmint oil is used in diffusers or applied topically after dilution to uplift mood and alleviate stress.

Herbal Baths: Spearmint leaves are added to bathwater for a soothing and aromatic bath that helps relax the muscles and clear the mind.

Decoctions: Boiling spearmint leaves in water creates a strong extract used for more intense therapeutic effects, particularly for digestive issues.

Syrups: Spearmint can be simmered with sugar and water to create a syrup, used to soothe sore throats and add flavor to beverages.

Gargles & Mouthwashes: A spearmint infusion is used as a gargle or mouthwash to freshen breath and promote oral health.

Powders: Dried spearmint leaves are ground into a powder for use in capsules or as a seasoning.

Juices: Spearmint leaves are juiced to make a refreshing drink that aids digestion and provides essential nutrients.

Culinary Uses: Spearmint is widely used in cooking for its flavor, added to salads, desserts, and beverages.

Ease to Grow: 2-3, Low Maintenance

Growing spearmint is quite straightforward, making it an excellent choice for novice gardeners. It thrives in well-draining soil and partial to full sunlight, requiring regular watering to keep the soil moist. Its vigorous growth habit means it can spread quickly, so it may be best to grow it in containers to contain its spread.

Spikenard

Also known as Nardostachys jatamansi, is a perennial herb native to the Himalayas. It has a long history of use in traditional medicine, particularly in Ayurvedic and Chinese practices. The plant's aromatic rhizomes are harvested for their medicinal and aromatic properties. Spikenard oil, derived from these rhizomes, is valued for its sedative, calming effects and is used in perfumery and aromatherapy.

Nervous System

Brain: Spikenard acts as a sedative, helping to calm the mind and alleviate symptoms of anxiety and stress. It is often used in traditional medicine to improve sleep quality and aid in the treatment of neurological disorders. The compounds in spikenard also have been studied for their potential to enhance cognitive function.

How to Grow Spikenard

- **Selecting the Right Variety:** Spikenard varieties are not commonly differentiated in the market. It is typically grown from root cuttings rather than seeds. Purchasing root cuttings from reputable nurseries or online stores specializing in medicinal herbs is recommended to ensure quality and authenticity.

- **Best Time to Plant Outdoors:** Plant spikenard root cuttings in early spring or fall. The cool temperatures help the roots establish without the stress of extreme heat.

- **Spacing Outdoor Plants:** Space plants or seeds about 18 to 24 inches apart to ensure adequate room for growth and airflow, reducing the risk of disease.

- **Container Use and Soil:** Spikenard prefers rich, well-drained soil with a good amount of organic matter. In containers, use a mix of garden soil, compost, and perlite or sand for drainage.

- **Sunlight and Location:** Prefers partial shade, with about 4 to 6 hours of sunlight daily. In regions with intense sun, provide afternoon shade to protect the plant.

- **Watering:** Keep the soil consistently moist but not waterlogged. Water when the top inch of soil feels dry to touch.

- **Feeding:** Fertilize with a balanced, slow-release organic fertilizer in early spring to support growth throughout the season.

- **Pruning and Maintenance:** Snip off dead flowers to promote more growth and prevent the plant from flowering too early, which can reduce the root's medicinal quality.

- **Pest and Disease Management:** Monitor for common garden pests and fungal diseases. Treat with organic pesticides or fungicides as needed, and ensure good air circulation to prevent disease.

- **Overwintering:** In colder climates, mulch around the base to protect roots from freezing temperatures.
- **Propagation:** Propagate by dividing root cuttings in the fall or early spring. Each section should have at least one growth bud.
- **Harvesting:** The roots are typically harvested in the fall of the third year after planting. Carefully dig around the plant and lift the root, cleaning it and drying for medicinal use.
- **Climate Considerations:** Thrives in cool, moist environments similar to its native habitat in the Himalayas. Not well-suited for extremely hot or dry climates.

How to Use Spikenard

Tinctures: Spikenard roots are soaked in alcohol to create tinctures, used for their calming and sedative properties to alleviate stress and promote sleep.

Decoctions: The dried roots are often simmered in water to make a decoction, helping to treat digestive issues and respiratory conditions.

Powders: Dried spikenard root is ground into a powder, used in capsule form or added to foods for its health benefits, including immune system support.

Ease to Grow: 5-7, Medium Maintenance

Growing spikenard requires some attention to ensure the right shade and soil conditions. It thrives in cooler climates and prefers a woodland setting, making it moderately challenging to cultivate in a typical garden. Regular watering and shade management are key to its successful growth and development.

Stevia

(Stevia Rebaudiana) is a natural sweetener and herb native to South America, known for its sweet leaves that have been used for hundreds of years to sweeten food and beverages. Stevia contains compounds called steviol glycosides, which are responsible for its sweetness and are calorie-free. This makes it a popular sugar substitute, especially for people with diabetes, as it does not raise blood sugar levels. Additionally, stevia has been studied for its antioxidant, anti-inflammatory, and antimicrobial properties, making it a subject of interest in both culinary and medicinal fields.

Endocrine System

Pancreas: Stevia aids in regulating blood sugar levels by stimulating insulin production, which can be beneficial for people with diabetes.

Digestive System

Stomach: Stevia has been shown to reduce gastric acidity and improve overall digestive health.

Cardiovascular System

Blood Pressure: Studies suggest that stevia can lower high blood pressure by acting as a vasodilator, expanding blood vessels and reducing the pressure on the cardiovascular system.

How to Grow Stevia

- **Selecting the Right Variety:** Stevia Rebaudiana is the most common variety for growing due to its high steviol glycoside content, which provides the sweetness. It's best to begin with starts or seedlings, as growing from seed can be challenging. These can be purchased online or from specialized nurseries that carry herb plants.
- **Best Time to Plant Outdoors:** Plant stevia in the spring after the danger of frost has passed. This timing allows the plant to establish itself during the warm months.
- **Spacing Outdoor Plants:** Space stevia plants about 18 inches apart to allow for adequate air circulation and growth, reducing the risk of disease.
- **Container Use and Soil:** Stevia thrives in well-draining soil with a neutral to slightly acidic pH. It can be grown in containers, using a high-quality potting mix that includes organic matter.
- **Sunlight and Location:** Stevia prefers full sun, requiring at least 6 to 8 hours of direct sunlight daily. In hot climates, some afternoon shade can prevent the plant from flowering too early.
- **Watering:** Water stevia regularly to keep the soil moist but not waterlogged, as the roots are prone to rot in overly wet conditions.
- **Feeding:** Apply a balanced, all-purpose fertilizer sparingly during the growing season to encourage growth without compromising the quality of the leaves.
- **Pruning and Maintenance:** Trim stevia to prevent it from flowering too early, which can reduce leaf sweetness. Regularly pinching off the tips encourages bushier growth.

- **Pest and Disease Management:** Stevia is relatively resistant to pests and diseases. However, monitor for common issues like aphids and address any fungal diseases promptly by improving air circulation and reducing leaf wetness.
- **Overwintering:** In colder climates, stevia should be overwintered indoors or treated as an annual. Dig up the plants before frost and pot them to keep indoors near a sunny window.
- **Propagation:** Stevia can be propagated from cuttings taken in late summer, which can then be overwintered indoors and replanted in the spring.
- **Harvesting:** Harvest stevia leaves before the plant flowers for the sweetest taste. Leaves can be picked throughout the growing season and dried for use as a natural sweetener.
- **Climate Considerations:** Stevia grows best in warm climates with consistent moisture. It can tolerate some heat but benefits from cooler nighttime temperatures and even moisture levels to thrive.

How to Use Stevia

Herbal Teas or Infusions: Leaves of stevia are soaked in hot water to create an herbal tea. This tea is naturally sweet, reducing the need for added sugars and offering a calorie-free alternative for sweetening beverages.

Tinctures: Stevia leaves are used to make tinctures, concentrating the sweet compounds in a liquid form that can be used to sweeten foods and drinks without the bulk of the leaves.

Powders: Dried stevia leaves can be ground into a fine powder used as a sugar substitute in cooking and baking, providing a sweet flavor without the calories or carbohydrates.

Culinary Uses: Stevia is primarily used in culinary applications as a natural sweetener. The leaves are used fresh or dried to sweeten teas, desserts, and other dishes, offering a healthful alternative to sugar.

Ease to Grow: 2-4, Low Maintenance

Stevia is considered low maintenance and relatively easy to grow. It prefers warm climates and well-drained soil but can also be grown in containers indoors under the right conditions. Regular watering and full sunlight are essential for optimal growth and leaf sweetness.

St. John's Wort

(Hypericum Perforatum) is a perennial herb known for its yellow flowers and medicinal properties. It's been used for centuries to treat various ailments. The plant contains active compounds like hypericin and hyperforin, which contribute to its therapeutic effects. St. John's Wort is particularly renowned for its impact on the nervous system, often used to alleviate depression, anxiety, and sleep disorders.

Nervous System

Brain: St. John's Wort influences neurotransmitter activity, enhancing mood and alleviating symptoms of depression and anxiety.
Nerves: It has nerve-regenerative properties, potentially aiding in the recovery of nerve tissue and reducing neuropathic pain.

Endocrine System

Thyroid gland: St. John's Wort can impact thyroid function, potentially normalizing some thyroid disorders by regulating hormonal activity.

How to Grow St. John's Wort

- **Selecting the Right Variety:** St. John's Wort (Hypericum Perforatum) is the most commonly used variety for medicinal purposes. Starting with seeds or starts is effective, but seeds require stratification to germinate. Purchase from reputable nurseries or online stores specializing in medicinal herbs.
- **Best Time to Plant Outdoors:** Plant in early spring or fall. Seeds should be sown in fall if they have undergone cold stratification (a period of cold or moist conditions to break dormancy and encourage germination).
- **Spacing Outdoor Plants:** Space plants or seeds about 18 inches apart to allow room for growth and air circulation.
- **Container Use and Soil:** Thrives in well-drained soil with a pH between 6.0 and 7.0. Suitable for container gardening, use pots with adequate drainage holes.
- **Sunlight and Location:** Prefers full sun to partial shade, needing around 6 to 8 hours of sunlight daily. Can use grow lights if natural sunlight is insufficient.
- **Watering:** Water regularly to keep the soil moist but not waterlogged. Reduce watering frequency once established.
- **Feeding:** Apply a balanced, slow-release fertilizer in the spring to support growth.
- **Pruning and Maintenance:** Snip off dead flowers to encourage more blooms and prevent the plant from flowering too early.

- **Pest and Disease Management:** Watch for common issues like powdery mildew or aphids. Treat with organic fungicides or insecticidal soap as needed.
- **Overwintering:** In colder climates, mulch around the base to protect roots in winter.
- **Propagation:** Easily propagated by seed, division, or cuttings in early spring or late summer.
- **Harvesting:** Harvest leaves and flowers in mid to late summer when in full bloom; these parts contain the active compounds. Dry them for medicinal use.
- **Climate Considerations:** Thrives in temperate climates with distinct seasons and well-distributed rainfall, avoiding extremely hot or cold conditions.

How to Use St. John's Wort

Herbal Teas or Infusions: Soak the dried flowers of St. John's Wort in hot water for about 10 minutes to make a calming tea that can alleviate mild depressive symptoms and soothe the nervous system.

Tinctures: The flowers and leaves are soaked in alcohol to extract the active compounds, creating a concentrated tincture that can be used to treat depression and anxiety.

Salves-Topical Applications: Infused oil made from St. John's Wort can be combined with beeswax to create salves or ointments that help heal wounds, burns, and soothe irritated skin.

Poultices: Crushed fresh or rehydrated dried flowers and leaves can be applied directly to the skin to relieve inflammation, bruises, and skin irritations.

Decoctions: Boiling the plant parts in water creates a strong decoction that can be used externally for its antiseptic and anti-inflammatory properties.

Syrups: The decoction can be mixed with honey or sugar to make a syrup that soothes sore throats and relieves respiratory issues.

Powders: Dried leaves and flowers are often ground into a fine powder that can be used for capsule supplements or as a wound-healing dust.

Ease to Grow: 3-5, Low Maintenance

St. John's Wort is a hardy perennial that grows easily in full sun and well-drained soil. It's low maintenance, self-seeding, and can spread rapidly, making it an easy plant to cultivate in a variety of garden settings.

Sweet Woodruff

Known scientifically as Galium Odoratum, is a fragrant, perennial herb native to Europe, North Africa, and Western Asia. It thrives in wooded areas, displaying white, star-shaped flowers in spring and early summer. Traditionally, Sweet Woodruff has been used for its medicinal and aromatic qualities. It contains coumarin, which imparts a fresh, hay-like scent, particularly when dried. Historically, it was used to flavor drinks, stuff mattresses, and repel insects.

Nervous System

Brain: Sweet Woodruff is known for its mild sedative effects, which can help alleviate stress and promote relaxation. It has been used to improve sleep quality and reduce anxiety, acting gently on the brain to induce calmness.

Digestive System

Stomach: Beneficial for soothing stomach ailments, including indigestion and heartburn. Its anti-inflammatory properties help to calm the lining of the stomach, easing discomfort associated with digestive issues.

How to Grow Sweet Woodruff

- **Selecting the Right Variety:** Sweet Woodruff (Galium Odoratum) is typically available in one main variety, known for its fragrant, white flowers and use as a ground cover. Start with nursery plants or seeds, available at garden centers or online. Prefers shady locations, making it ideal for woodland gardens.
- **Best Time to Plant Outdoors:** Plant in early spring or fall. This timing allows the plant to establish roots before extreme weather conditions, either the summer heat or winter cold.
- **Spacing Outdoor Plants:** Space plants or seeds about 12 inches apart to allow for spreading and adequate air circulation, reducing the risk of fungal diseases.
- **Container Use and Soil:** Thrives in moist, well-drained soil rich in organic matter. Suitable for container gardening if the pot provides enough space for root expansion and has good drainage.
- **Sunlight and Location:** Prefers partial to full shade, ideal under trees or in shaded garden corners. Can tolerate a few hours of morning sun but should be protected from harsh afternoon light.

- **Watering:** Keep the soil consistently moist, especially during dry spells. Sweet Woodruff prefers a damp environment but is not tolerant of waterlogged conditions.
- **Feeding:** Apply a balanced, slow-release fertilizer in early spring to support growth, especially if the soil is not rich in organic matter.
- **Pruning and Maintenance:** Snip off dead flowers to promote bushier growth and prevent the plant from flowering too early. Regularly check for and remove any yellow or damaged leaves to keep the plant healthy.
- **Pest and Disease Management:** Generally pest-resistant, but watch for signs of slug or snail damage. Fungal diseases can occur in overly wet conditions; ensure good soil drainage and air circulation.
- **Overwintering:** Hardy in most climates and typically survives winter without special care. Mulch around the base in very cold regions to protect the roots.
- **Propagation:** Easily propagated by division in spring or autumn. Separate clumps and replant to increase coverage or create new plantings.
- **Harvesting:** Leaves and flowers can be harvested just before the plant blooms, usually in late spring or early summer. Used fresh or dried for their aromatic properties and in herbal blends.
- **Climate Considerations:** Thrives in temperate climates with cool, moist conditions. Not suited for extremely hot and dry environments, prefers areas with seasonal changes.

How to Use Sweet Woodruff

Herbal Teas or Infusions: Sweet Woodruff leaves are soaked in hot water to create a fragrant tea, often consumed for its mild sedative effects and to aid digestion.

Tinctures: The leaves and flowers are soaked in alcohol to extract their active compounds, creating a tincture that is used for its therapeutic properties.

Culinary Uses: Sweet Woodruff is used to flavor drinks, jellies, and syrups. It imparts a sweet, hay-like taste and is especially popular in German May wine.

Ease to Grow: 2-3, Low Maintenance

Sweet Woodruff is an undemanding plant that thrives in shady, moist environments. Once established, it requires minimal care, spreading easily to form a dense ground cover. Its sweet-smelling flowers and leaves are valued in herbal teas and culinary dishes, making it a delightful addition to any garden.

Tarragon

Known scientifically as Artemisia Dracunculus, is a perennial herb distinguished by its slender, aromatic leaves. Originating in Eurasia, tarragon plays a significant role in various culinary traditions, particularly in French cuisine, where it's a component of the classic "fines herbes" blend. Beyond its culinary use, tarragon has been utilized historically for medicinal purposes, thanks to its various health-promoting properties.

Digestive System

Stomach: Tarragon can stimulate the production of digestive juices, which helps improve digestion and appetite.

Intestines: It is known to aid in relieving common digestive ailments, such as upset stomach and irritable bowel syndrome.

Nervous System

Brain: Tarragon contains compounds that may positively affect mood and reduce anxiety.

Nerves: It is used in herbal medicine to help calm the nerves and alleviate stress-related symptoms.

Cardiovascular System

Heart: Tarragon is believed to improve heart health by influencing blood circulation and maintaining healthy blood pressure levels.

Muscular System

Muscles: Tarragon oil is sometimes used to relieve muscle spasms and pain.

How to Grow Tarragon

- **Selecting the Right Variety:** French Tarragon is the preferred variety for culinary use, offering a more refined flavor than Russian or Mexican tarragon. French tarragon doesn't produce viable seeds, so it's best to purchase starter plants from a nursery or garden center.
- **Best Time to Plant Outdoors:** Plant tarragon in early spring after the last frost, ensuring a long growing season for the plant to establish.

- **Spacing Outdoor Plants:** Space tarragon plants about 18 to 24 inches apart to allow for adequate air circulation and growth.
- **Container Use and Soil:** Tarragon thrives in well-draining soil and can be grown in containers. Use a high-quality potting mix to ensure good drainage and avoid waterlogging.
- **Sunlight and Location:** Tarragon requires full sun, at least 6 hours of direct sunlight per day. If growing indoors, use a grow light to provide sufficient light intensity.
- **Watering:** Water tarragon regularly, allowing the soil to dry out slightly between waterings. Overwatering can lead to root rot.
- **Feeding:** Fertilize tarragon sparingly, as too much fertilizer can reduce the flavor of the leaves. A light application of a balanced, organic fertilizer in the spring is sufficient.
- **Pruning and Maintenance:** Snip off dead flowers to prevent the plant from flowering too early and to encourage bushier growth.
- **Pest and Disease Management:** Watch for common pests like aphids. Tarragon can be susceptible to root rot; ensure good drainage and avoid overwatering to prevent this.
- **Overwintering:** In colder climates, mulch around the base of the plant to protect it from freezing temperatures or grow in containers that can be moved indoors.
- **Propagation:** Propagate tarragon by root division or stem cuttings in spring or early summer to ensure vigorous growth.
- **Harvesting:** Harvest tarragon leaves in the morning when the essential oil content is highest. Leaves can be harvested throughout the growing season as needed.

- **Climate Considerations:** Tarragon grows best in areas with cool springs and autumns, warm summers, and moderate winters. It prefers a climate that avoids extreme heat or cold.

How to Use Tarragon

Herbal Teas or Infusions: Tarragon leaves can be soaked in hot water to create an herbal tea, offering a unique, mildly bittersweet flavor and potential digestive benefits.

Tinctures: The leaves and stems of tarragon can be used to make tinctures, which may aid in digestion and promote appetite.

Culinary Uses: Tarragon is widely used in cooking, especially in French cuisine, for flavoring a variety of dishes including sauces, salads, and meats. Its leaves are known for their distinctive anise-like flavor.

Ease to Grow: 3-5, Medium Maintenance

Tarragon is moderately easy to grow, requiring well-drained soil, plenty of sunlight, and regular watering. It thrives in temperate climates and can be grown in both gardens and containers.

Thyme

(Thymus vulgaris) is a perennial herb known for its aromatic leaves, which are used both in culinary and medicinal applications.

Originating in the Mediterranean region, thyme has been valued since ancient times for its therapeutic properties. It's a small, shrub-like plant with a woody stem, small leaves, and flowers that can range in color from white to purple. Thyme is rich in essential oils, thymol being one of the most significant, which contributes to its antiseptic and antibacterial qualities.

Respiratory System

Lungs: Thyme acts as an expectorant, helping to clear mucus from the lungs and relieve coughing.

Bronchi: It has antispasmodic properties, reducing spasms and aiding in the treatment of bronchitis and asthma.

Digestive System

Stomach: Thyme promotes digestion, reduces gas, and alleviates stomach discomfort.

Intestines: It has antimicrobial properties that can help in managing gastrointestinal infections.

Immune System

General Immune Support: Thyme supports the immune system due to its high antioxidant content, helping to fight off infections.

Skin and Integumentary System

Skin: Thyme's antiseptic and anti-inflammatory properties make it beneficial for treating skin conditions, aiding in wound healing and reducing inflammation.

How to Grow Thyme

- **Selecting the Right Variety:** Common thyme (Thymus Vulgaris) is most popular for culinary use, with varieties like lemon thyme (Thymus Citriodorus) offering unique flavors. Starting with young plants from a nursery is often easier and faster than growing from seeds.

- **Best Time to Plant Outdoors:** Early spring, after the last frost, is the best time to plant thyme outdoors, allowing the plant to establish before the hot summer.
- **Spacing Outdoor Plants:** Space thyme plants about 9 to 12 inches apart to ensure adequate air circulation and room for growth.
- **Container Use and Soil:** Thyme thrives in well-draining soil and can be grown in containers. Use a potting mix designed for succulents or add sand to improve drainage.
- **Sunlight and Location:** Thyme requires full sun, at least 6 hours of direct sunlight daily. If growing indoors, use a full-spectrum grow light to supplement light needs.
- **Watering:** Water thyme when the soil is dry to the touch. Overwatering can lead to root rot, so ensure the soil drains well.
- **Feeding:** Feed thyme sparingly; too much fertilizer can dilute the flavor of the leaves. A light application of organic fertilizer in the spring is sufficient.
- **Pruning and Maintenance:** Snip off dead flowers to encourage bushier growth and prevent the plant from flowering too early.
- **Pest and Disease Management:** Keep an eye out for fungal diseases, especially in humid conditions. Good air circulation and well-draining soil are critical for prevention.
- **Overwintering:** In colder climates, protect outdoor thyme with mulch or bring containers indoors to avoid freezing.
- **Propagation:** Propagate thyme by division or stem cuttings in the spring or early summer to ensure healthy new plants.

- **Harvesting:** Harvest thyme leaves just before the plant flowers for the best flavor, cutting stems in the morning when essential oils are concentrated.
- **Climate Considerations:** Thyme prefers a temperate climate with a balance of sunny and cool, dry periods. It tolerates cold better than excessive moisture or heat.

How to Use Thyme

Herbal Teas or Infusions: Thyme leaves can be soaked in hot water to create a herbal tea that is beneficial for treating coughs and sore throats due to its antimicrobial properties.

Tinctures: Thyme is used in tinctures to extract its essential oils, which are helpful for respiratory and digestive health.

Salves-Topical Applications: Thyme can be infused into salves or ointments to apply topically, aiding in the healing of skin infections and inflammations.

Decoctions: A decoction of thyme can be made by boiling the herb to concentrate its beneficial compounds, used for respiratory ailments.

Syrups: Thyme is often included in herbal syrups for cough and sore throat relief due to its expectorant properties.

Gargles & Mouthwashes: A thyme infusion can be used as a gargle or mouthwash to treat throat infections and improve oral health.

Culinary Uses: Thyme is extensively used in cooking for flavoring dishes, including meats, soups, and sauces, and is valued for its aromatic and preservative qualities.

Ease to Grow: 2-4, Low Maintenance

Thyme is easy to grow, requiring minimal care. It prefers well-drained soil and plenty of sunlight. With its drought-resistant nature, thyme thrives in various environments, making it a low-maintenance choice.

Turmeric

(Curcuma Longa) is a perennial plant native to Southeast Asia, widely known for its vibrant yellow-orange rhizome. Used extensively in cooking, particularly in Indian cuisine, turmeric also has a long history in traditional medicine. Its active compound, curcumin, is credited with numerous health benefits, including anti-inflammatory, antioxidant, and antimicrobial properties. Turmeric is commonly used in powdered form but is also available as fresh root, supplements, and extracts.

Digestive System

Stomach: Turmeric helps to stimulate digestion and can relieve bloating and gas.

Intestines: It supports intestinal health by promoting beneficial gut flora and reducing inflammation.

Immune System

General Immune Support: Turmeric strengthens the immune system due to its antioxidant properties, helping your body fight off infections.

Skin and Integumentary System

Skin: Its anti-inflammatory and antimicrobial properties make turmeric beneficial in treating skin conditions like eczema, psoriasis, and acne.

Cardiovascular System

Blood Vessels: Turmeric aids in improving circulation and reducing cholesterol levels, which can help prevent heart disease.

Endocrine System

Pancreas: It may help regulate insulin levels and improve glucose control, beneficial for managing diabetes.

Skeletal System

Bones and Joints: Turmeric is known for its effectiveness in reducing joint pain and inflammation, commonly used in conditions like arthritis.

How to Grow Turmeric

- **Selecting the Right Variety:** The most common variety of turmeric used for both culinary and medicinal purposes is Curcuma Longa. Turmeric is typically grown from rhizomes (root cuttings) rather than seeds, as it's easier and faster. Rhizomes can be purchased online or from a garden center specializing in tropical plants.
- **Best Time to Plant Outdoors:** The best time to plant turmeric is in the spring after the risk of frost has passed, as it requires a long, warm growing season to mature.
- **Spacing Outdoor Plants:** Plant turmeric rhizomes about 12 to 18 inches apart to allow enough space for the plants to grow.
- **Container Use and Soil:** Turmeric can be grown in containers using well-draining, fertile soil rich in organic matter. It prefers slightly acidic to neutral pH.

- **Sunlight and Location:** Turmeric needs warm conditions and partial shade or indirect sunlight. If growing indoors, use grow lights to simulate warm conditions with adequate light.
- **Watering:** Keep the soil moist but not waterlogged. Turmeric requires consistent watering, especially during the warmer months of its growth period.
- **Feeding:** Use a balanced, organic fertilizer every couple of months to provide the nutrients turmeric needs for growth.
- **Pruning and Maintenance:** There is little need for pruning, but remove any yellow or dead leaves to keep the plant healthy.
- **Pest and Disease Management:** Watch for signs of fungal diseases like leaf spot, which appears as brown spots on leaves. Improve air circulation and reduce watering to manage these issues.
- **Overwintering:** In cooler climates, turmeric should be overwintered indoors or in a greenhouse to protect it from cold temperatures.
- **Propagation:** Turmeric is propagated from rhizomes. Each piece of rhizome planted will produce a new plant.
- **Harvesting:** Turmeric roots are ready to harvest after 8-10 months when the leaves and stem start to brown and dry. The roots are dug up, and both fresh and dried rhizomes have health benefits.
- **Climate Considerations:** Turmeric thrives in warm, humid climates similar to its native Southeast Asia, where there is consistent warmth and high humidity.

How to Use Turmeric

Herbal Teas or Infusions: Turmeric root can be soaked in hot water to make a tea that is beneficial for its anti-inflammatory and antioxidant properties.

Tinctures: Turmeric tincture is used in its concentrated form to support immune function and reduce inflammation.

Salves-Topical Applications: Turmeric can be used in creams and ointments for its anti-inflammatory and antibacterial properties, aiding in wound healing and skin care.

Decoctions: A turmeric decoction, boiled to concentrate its compounds, can be consumed for digestive health and to reduce inflammation.

Powders: Turmeric powder is commonly used for its health benefits, including anti-inflammatory, antioxidant, and metabolic health support.

Juices: Turmeric juice, often combined with other fruits or vegetables, is consumed for its detoxifying and anti-inflammatory benefits.

Culinary Uses: Turmeric is widely used in cooking for its flavor and color, most notably in curries, and has health benefits such as anti-inflammatory and antioxidant properties.

Ease to Grow: 5-7, Medium Maintenance

Turmeric is moderately easy to grow with the right conditions, needing a warm, humid climate and careful attention to watering and soil quality to prevent root rot.

Uva Ursi

Also known as bearberry, is a small evergreen shrub whose leaves are used in herbal medicine. It thrives in cooler climates across North America, Europe, and Asia. The plant produces small, leathery leaves and bright red berries, but it's the leaves that are most valued for their medicinal properties. They contain compounds like arbutin, which is converted into hydroquinone in the body, providing antiseptic properties. Traditionally, Uva Ursi has been used to treat urinary tract infections, kidney stones, and other ailments related to the urinary system.

Urinary System

Kidneys: Uva Ursi is known to have diuretic properties, aiding in the flushing of kidneys and potentially helping to remove kidney stones.
Bladder: Its antiseptic qualities can help in treating and preventing urinary tract infections by reducing bacteria in the bladder.
Urethra: Uva Ursi's compounds soothe inflammation and can aid in the healing of urethral irritations.

How to Grow Uva Ursi

- **Selecting the Right Variety:** Uva Ursi, or bearberry, has several varieties, but the most commonly used for medicinal purposes is Arctostaphylos uva-ursi. Starting from seeds or nursery-bought plants is common. Seeds can be slow to germinate, so purchasing young plants from a reputable nursery might be preferable for faster establishment.

- **Best Time to Plant Outdoors:** Early spring or fall is the best time to plant Uva Ursi outdoors, when the temperature is cooler and the plant can establish itself without the stress of extreme heat.
- **Spacing Outdoor Plants:** Space plants or seeds about 12 inches apart to ensure enough room for growth and air circulation.
- **Container Use and Soil:** Uva Ursi prefers well-drained, sandy or loamy soil with a slightly acidic pH. It can be grown in containers if the soil is well-aerated and not overly rich.
- **Sunlight and Location:** This plant thrives in full sun to partial shade. It requires around 6 to 8 hours of sunlight daily. If grown under artificial light, use LED grow lights to mimic natural sunlight conditions.
- **Watering:** Water regularly to keep the soil moist but not waterlogged. Uva Ursi does not tolerate overwatering well, so ensure good drainage.
- **Feeding:** Fertilize sparingly, as Uva Ursi prefers nutrient-poor soil. A light application of a balanced, slow-release fertilizer in the spring is sufficient.
- **Pruning and Maintenance:** Snip off dead flowers to encourage healthy growth and prevent the plant from putting energy into seed production.
- **Pest and Disease Management:** Uva Ursi is relatively disease-resistant but watch for signs of leaf spot or root rot, which appear as discolored or wilting leaves. Treat with fungicides and ensure good soil drainage to prevent these issues.

- **Overwintering:** In colder climates, apply a layer of mulch around the base of the plant to protect it from freezing temperatures.
- **Propagation:** Propagate by seed in autumn or by cuttings in late spring to early summer. Root division can also be done in early spring or fall.
- **Harvesting:** The leaves of Uva Ursi can be harvested anytime during the growing season, but the best time is in summer when the concentrations of active compounds are highest. Dry the leaves for use in teas or extracts.
- **Climate Considerations:** Uva Ursi is best suited for cool, temperate climates with well-drained soils. It can tolerate cold temperatures well, making it suitable for northern regions.

How to Use Uva Ursi

Herbal Teas or Infusions: Uva Ursi leaves are soaked in hot water to create a tea that is commonly used to support urinary tract health and help with inflammation.

Tinctures: The leaves of Uva Ursi are soaked in alcohol to extract their beneficial compounds, creating a tincture used for its antiseptic and diuretic properties.

Salves-Topical Applications: Uva Ursi can be incorporated into salves, creams, or ointments to apply topically, helping to treat skin irritations and promote healing.

Decoctions: Leaves are simmered in water for an extended period to make a strong decoction, used traditionally for urinary tract support and as a mild diuretic.

Powders: Dried Uva Ursi leaves can be ground into a powder, which is used for its health benefits, especially related to urinary tract health.

Ease to Grow: 3-6, Medium Maintenance

Uva Ursi is adaptable to various environments but requires specific soil conditions and shade levels, making it moderately easy to grow with some attention to detail.

Valerian

Scientifically known as Valeriana Officinalis, is a perennial flowering plant native to Europe and Asia. It has sweetly scented pink or white flowers and is primarily cultivated for its roots. Valerian root has been used in traditional medicine for centuries, mainly for its sedative and calming effects. It is commonly used to treat sleep disorders, anxiety, and psychological stress. The active compounds in valerian, such as valerenic acid, interact with the GABA (gamma-aminobutyric acid) neurotransmitter system in the brain, which helps to reduce nervous tension and promote relaxation.

Nervous System

Central Nervous System: Valerian is known for its calming effects on the central nervous system, promoting relaxation and reducing anxiety.

Peripheral Nervous System: It may also help alleviate symptoms of nervous tension and stress.

Muscular System

Smooth Muscles: Valerian has been observed to relax smooth muscles, potentially aiding in the relief of muscle spasms and tension.

How to Grow Valerian

- **Selecting the Right Variety:** Valerian Officinalis is the most commonly cultivated variety for medicinal use. Starting from seeds or plant divisions is common. Seeds can be purchased from garden centers or online. They have a short viability period, so fresh seeds are preferable.
- **Best Time to Plant Outdoors:** Plant valerian in early spring or fall. The cooler temperatures help the seeds to germinate more effectively.
- **Spacing Outdoor Plants:** Space plants or seeds about 1 to 2 feet apart to ensure they have enough room to grow and spread.
- **Container Use and Soil:** Valerian grows well in containers with well-draining soil rich in organic matter. It prefers a neutral to slightly acidic pH.
- **Sunlight and Location:** Valerian requires full sun to partial shade, with around 6 to 8 hours of sunlight daily. If using artificial light, full-spectrum LED lights are suitable.
- **Watering:** Keep the soil consistently moist but not waterlogged. Valerian needs regular watering, especially during dry periods.
- **Feeding:** Apply a balanced, organic fertilizer in the spring to support growth throughout the season.
- **Pruning and Maintenance:** Snip off dead flowers to encourage more growth and prevent the plant from using energy to produce seeds.

- **Pest and Disease Management:** Monitor for common pests like aphids and treat with organic insecticides. Root rot can occur in overly wet conditions, so ensure good drainage.
- **Overwintering:** In colder climates, mulch around the base of the plant to protect it from freezing temperatures.
- **Propagation:** Propagate by seed in the fall or by root division in the spring or fall. Dividing the plants every 3 to 4 years can rejuvenate them and prevent overcrowding.
- **Harvesting:** The roots are the most valuable part and can be harvested in the fall of the second year. Dig up the roots carefully, clean them, and then dry for medicinal use.
- **Climate Considerations:** Valerian prefers climates with distinct seasons and does well in areas with cool, moist summers and cold winters.

How to Use Valerian

Herbal Teas or Infusions: Valerian root is cut into pieces and soaked in hot water to make a tea, commonly used for its sedative properties to improve sleep and reduce anxiety.

Tinctures: The roots are soaked in alcohol to create a tincture, best taken in small doses to help with sleep and reduce stress.

Decoctions: A decoction is made by boiling valerian root, concentrating its active compounds, and is used to aid sleep and soothe nervous tension.

Powders: The dried root can be ground into a powder, which is then used in capsules or mixed into beverages to promote relaxation and improve sleep quality.

Ease to Grow: 3-5, Low Maintenance

Valerian is relatively easy to grow, adaptable to various soil types, and requires minimal maintenance, making it great for beginners.

Vervain

Scientifically known as Verbena Officinalis, is an herbaceous plant with a long history of use in traditional medicine and folklore. It is native to Europe but has been naturalized in various regions worldwide. Vervain is valued for its potential health benefits and is often used in herbal preparations such as teas, tinctures, and extracts.

Nervous System

Central Nervous System: Vervain is believed to have calming properties that can help soothe the central nervous system, promoting relaxation and reducing symptoms of anxiety or stress.

Peripheral Nervous System: It may also have a beneficial effect on the peripheral nervous system, helping to alleviate tension and nervousness.

Muscular System

Muscles: Vervain is thought to aid in the relaxation of smooth muscles, which can be beneficial for relieving muscle tension and spasms, particularly in the digestive tract.

How to Grow Vervain

- **Selecting the Right Variety:** Vervain (Verbena Officinalis) is the common variety used for medicinal purposes, but there are ornamental types too, like Verbena Bonariensis. Starting with seeds is usually preferred as it allows for a wider selection of varieties. Seeds or starts can be purchased from nurseries, garden centers, or online retailers specializing in medicinal herbs.

- **Best Time to Plant Outdoors:** Plant vervain seeds or starts in the spring after the last frost, as this gives the plant time to establish itself during the warmer months.
- **Spacing Outdoor Plants:** Space vervain plants or seeds about 12 to 18 inches apart. This allows enough room for each plant to grow and receive adequate sunlight and air circulation.
- **Container Use and Soil:** Vervain grows well in containers using well-draining soil. For outdoor and pot cultivation, a loamy or sandy soil enriched with organic matter is ideal, mimicking its natural growing conditions.
- **Sunlight and Location:** Vervain needs full sun, at least 6 to 8 hours of direct sunlight daily. If using artificial lighting, LED grow lights set for 14-16 hours a day can mimic these conditions.
- **Watering:** Water vervain regularly to keep the soil moist but not waterlogged. The plant prefers consistent moisture, especially during hot, dry periods.
- **Feeding:** Fertilize vervain lightly in the spring with a balanced, slow-release fertilizer to support growth throughout the flowering period.
- **Pruning and Maintenance:** Snip off dead flowers to promote continuous blooming and prevent the plant from expending energy on seed production.
- **Pest and Disease Management:** Vervain is susceptible to powdery mildew and rust. Look for white powdery spots or rust-colored patches on leaves. Treat with fungicides or natural remedies like neem oil and ensure good air circulation.

- **Overwintering:** In colder climates, mulch around the base to protect roots from freezing or pot the plant and bring indoors during winter.
- **Propagation:** Propagate vervain by seed, cuttings, or division in early spring or autumn. This helps to maintain healthy, vigorous plants.
- **Harvesting:** Harvest vervain leaves and flowers during the blooming season, usually in summer, as these parts are rich in beneficial compounds. Cut the stems in the morning after dew has evaporated for the best potency.
- **Climate Considerations:** Vervain thrives in climates where it can receive plenty of sunlight and has a distinct growing season, with warm summers and cool winters. It can adapt to a range of conditions but prefers a temperate climate.

How to Use Vervain

- **Herbal Teas or Infusions:** Soak dried vervain leaves in hot water for 5-10 minutes to create a soothing herbal tea.
- **Tinctures:** Prepare a tincture by macerating vervain leaves in alcohol for several weeks, then strain to extract its medicinal properties.
- **Salves-Topical Applications:** Create a healing salve with infused vervain oil, suitable for topical use on minor cuts and bruises.
- **Compresses:** Make a compress with vervain-infused water to alleviate muscle soreness or reduce inflammation.
- **Aromatherapy & Essential Oils:** Use vervain essential oil in a diffuser for aromatherapy benefits, or dilute it for direct application on pulse points.

- **Herbal Baths:** Enhance your bath experience by adding dried vervain leaves to the water for a relaxing herbal soak.
- **Steam Inhalation:** Infuse boiling water with vervain leaves to create a steam inhalation that helps clear sinus congestion.
- **Decoctions:** Boil vervain roots in water to create a decoction for internal use, offering potential health benefits.
- **Syrups:** Combine vervain-infused water with sweetener to make a syrup, ideal for soothing coughs and sore throats.
- **Gargles & Mouthwashes:** Use vervain-infused water as a gargle or mouthwash for oral hygiene and freshness.
- **Powders:** Grind dried vervain leaves into a powder for encapsulation or incorporation into various recipes.
- **Juices:** Extract juice from fresh vervain leaves to add a nutritious boost to beverages or culinary creations.
- **Culinary Uses:** Incorporate fresh or dried vervain leaves into soups, stews, or herbal infusions for added flavor and potential health benefits.

Ease to Grow: 5-7, Medium Maintenance

Vervain falls into the category of plants with moderate ease of cultivation, requiring regular attention and care but not overly demanding. It's suitable for gardeners with some experience and a willingness to provide consistent watering, proper soil conditions, and occasional pruning or maintenance tasks. While it doesn't require expert-level skills, beginners may find it slightly challenging compared to low-maintenance plants.

Watercress

(Nasturtium Officinale) is a fast-growing, aquatic or semi-aquatic perennial plant known for its peppery-flavored leaves. It is rich in vitamins A, C, and K, and contains significant amounts of calcium, iron, and folate. Traditionally, watercress has been used for its medicinal properties, including boosting immunity, preventing chronic diseases, and serving as a natural diuretic. It is also known for its antioxidant properties, which help fight free radicals and support overall health.

Digestive System

Stomach: Watercress aids in digestion by stimulating the release of digestive enzymes, helping to soothe stomach upsets and improve digestion.

Respiratory System

Lungs: Watercress has expectorant properties, helping to clear congestion in the lungs and alleviate symptoms of respiratory conditions like bronchitis.

Cardiovascular System

Blood vessels: The high levels of antioxidants and

anti-inflammatory compounds in watercress can help lower blood pressure and reduce the risk of heart disease.

Immune System

General Immunity: The high vitamin C content in watercress boosts the immune system, enhancing the body's ability to fight off infections and diseases.

Skin and Integumentary System

Skin: The nutrients in watercress, especially vitamins A and C, promote healthy skin by enhancing skin texture and elasticity, and helping to prevent skin aging and damage.

How to Grow Watercress

- **Selecting the Right Variety:** Common watercress (Nasturtium Officinale) is the most widely cultivated variety, known for its peppery flavor and health benefits. Seeds or starter plants can be purchased from garden centers or online retailers. Starting from seeds is cost-effective, while starter plants can provide a quicker harvest.
- **Best Time to Plant Outdoors:** Early spring is the best time to plant watercress outdoors when the risk of frost has passed and the water temperatures are still cool.
- **Spacing Outdoor Plants:** Space watercress plants or seeds about 8 to 10 inches apart to allow room for growth and reduce overcrowding, which can lead to pest and disease issues.
- **Container Use and Soil:** Watercress grows best in consistently wet, boggy soil conditions. It can be grown in containers if they are kept in trays of water or a water-retentive soil mix.

- **Sunlight and Location:** Watercress prefers partial shade but can tolerate full sun if kept in constantly moist soil. In regions with hot summers, provide afternoon shade to prevent wilting.
- **Watering:** Maintain consistently moist or shallow standing water for watercress. The plant's natural habitat is along streams and water bodies, so replicate these conditions as closely as possible.
- **Feeding:** Fertilize watercress lightly with a liquid plant food every 4 to 6 weeks during the growing season to support its rapid growth.
- **Pruning and Maintenance:** Regularly harvest leaves to encourage new growth and prevent the plant from flowering too early, which can affect the taste.
- **Pest and Disease Management:** Keep an eye out for common pests like aphids and snails. Control pests manually or with organic pesticides, and ensure good water quality to prevent diseases.
- **Overwintering:** Watercress can be overwintered in milder climates by ensuring it remains in water and is protected from freezing temperatures.
- **Propagation:** Watercress can be propagated by stem cuttings placed in water, where they quickly root and can be transplanted.
- **Harvesting:** Harvest watercress leaves and stems as needed, cutting them near the base. The plant continues to grow, providing a continuous supply. Watercress is best harvested before it flowers for optimal flavor.
- **Climate Considerations:** Watercress grows best in cool, moist climates. It thrives in temperatures between 50-70°F and can be grown year-round in temperate regions with adequate water supply.

How to Use Watercress

Herbal Teas or Infusions: Watercress leaves and stems can be soaked in hot water to create an herbal tea, offering a peppery flavor and health benefits like improved respiratory function and digestion.

Decoctions: Boiling watercress in water makes a strong decoction used traditionally to treat kidney and respiratory ailments due to its diuretic and expectorant properties.

Juices: Watercress can be juiced alone or with other vegetables and fruits to create a nutrient-rich drink, high in vitamins and antioxidants, promoting overall health.

Culinary Uses: Watercress is extensively used in salads, sandwiches, soups, and as a garnish due to its peppery flavor, adding both nutritional and culinary value to dishes.

Ease to Grow: 3-5, Low Maintenance

Watercress is a low-maintenance plant that grows quickly in wet, aquatic environments. It requires consistent moisture and can be grown in shallow water or very moist soil. With its ability to thrive in cool to moderate climates and its adaptability to various water conditions, watercress is an accessible plant for beginner gardeners.

White Willow Bark

Comes from the white willow tree, scientifically known as Salix Alba. This tree is native to Europe and Central Asia but has been widely cultivated in other regions for its medicinal properties. The bark contains salicin, a compound that the body converts into salicylic acid, which is the precursor to aspirin. Traditionally, white willow bark has been used for its pain-relieving, anti-inflammatory, and fever-reducing properties. It has a long history in herbal medicine for treating various ailments, especially those involving pain and inflammation.

Nervous System

Pain perception: White Willow Bark is known to reduce pain by inhibiting the production of certain chemicals in the body that signal pain.

Cardiovascular System

Blood vessels: It helps in maintaining cardiovascular health by promoting healthy blood circulation and potentially reducing the risk of clot formation.

Muscular System

Muscles: The anti-inflammatory properties of white willow bark can help in relieving muscle aches and pains.

Skeletal System

Joints: Commonly used to alleviate joint pain and reduce inflammation associated with conditions like arthritis.

How to Grow White Willow Bark

- **Selecting the Right Variety:** The most common variety for medicinal use is Salix Alba (White Willow). It can be grown from cuttings or seeds, with cuttings being the preferred method for faster growth. Purchase these from nurseries or online stores specializing in medicinal plants.
- **Best Time to Plant Outdoors:** Early spring is the best time to plant willow cuttings directly into the ground.
- **Spacing Outdoor Plants:** Space willow trees at least 20 feet apart to allow for their wide-reaching root systems and canopy growth.
- **Container Use and Soil:** While white willow prefers being planted in the ground due to its large size, it can grow in large containers with well-draining soil initially before being transplanted outdoors.
- **Sunlight and Location:** White willow trees need full sun to partial shade, requiring at least 6 hours of sunlight daily. They do not need artificial lighting if planted outdoors.
- **Watering:** Willow trees love moist soil, so water them regularly to keep the soil constantly wet, especially during dry periods.
- **Feeding:** Apply a balanced fertilizer in early spring to support growth, but avoid over-fertilizing as willows are generally low-maintenance in nutrient requirements.

- **Pruning and Maintenance:** Prune in late winter to remove dead branches and shape the tree. Snip off dead flowers to maintain health and appearance.
- **Pest and Disease Management:** Watch for willow beetle or aphid infestations and treat with appropriate insecticides. Fungal diseases like scab or rust can be managed with fungicides and by ensuring good air circulation.
- **Overwintering:** White willow is hardy and can tolerate cold winters. No special overwintering measures are required.
- **Propagation:** Propagate by taking cuttings in late winter or early spring and planting them directly in moist soil.
- **Harvesting:** The bark is harvested in the spring from young branches or trunks. Peel the bark carefully and dry it for medicinal use, such as for making tinctures or teas.

- **Climate Considerations:** White willow thrives in cool to temperate climates with consistent moisture. It is well-suited for areas with wet soils and can tolerate occasional flooding.

How to Use White Willow Bark

Herbal Teas or Infusions: The bark can be cut into small pieces and soaked in boiling water to make an infusion, often used for pain relief and anti-inflammatory purposes.

Tinctures: White Willow Bark is soaked in alcohol to create a tincture, which can be used to alleviate pain, inflammation, and fevers.

Salves-Topical Applications: The bark is used in salves, creams, or ointments for topical application to relieve pain and reduce inflammation in areas like muscles and joints.

Decoctions: A strong decoction is made by simmering the bark in water, used to treat aches, pains, and to reduce fever.

Powders: The dried bark is ground into a powder, which can be used in capsules or mixed with liquids for consumption to utilize its pain-relieving and anti-inflammatory effects.

Ease to Grow: 2-4, Low Maintenance

White Willow is relatively easy to grow, requiring minimal care once established, and is adaptable to various environmental conditions.

Wild Yam

Scientifically known as Dioscorea Villosa, is a perennial vine native to North America. It's known for its tuberous roots, which have been used in traditional medicine for centuries. Wild yam contains compounds like diosgenin, which is thought to contribute to its medicinal properties. It has been traditionally used to treat a range of ailments, including menstrual pain, digestive issues, and to ease childbirth. The plant is also used in alternative medicine as a natural precursor to various steroid hormones.

Reproductive System

Ovaries: Wild Yam is believed to support ovarian health and may help balance hormone levels, potentially easing menstrual cramps and menopausal symptoms.

Digestive System

Stomach: It is used to help alleviate digestive discomfort, such as cramps and spasms, by relaxing smooth muscles in the digestive tract.

Endocrine System

Hormones: Wild Yam influences the production of various hormones, aiding in the balance and regulation of hormonal activities in the body.

How to Grow Wild Yam

- **Selecting the Right Variety:** Dioscorea Villosa (Wild Yam) is the most commonly used variety for medicinal purposes. It is typically propagated from tubers (underground stems) rather than seeds. Tubers or starter plants can be purchased from herbal nurseries or online stores specializing in medicinal plants.

- **Best Time to Plant Outdoors:** Spring is the best time to plant wild yam tubers, after the risk of frost has passed.

- **Spacing Outdoor Plants:** Space plants or tubers about 8 to 10 feet apart to accommodate their sprawling growth and extensive root systems.

- **Container Use and Soil:** Wild yam can be grown in large containers with well-draining, loamy soil. Ensure the pot has adequate drainage holes to prevent waterlogging.

- **Sunlight and Location:** Prefers partial shade but can tolerate full sun. In areas with intense sunlight, provide some afternoon shade to prevent overheating. Artificial lighting is not typically necessary.

- **Watering:** Water regularly to keep the soil consistently moist but not waterlogged. Wild yam roots do not tolerate drought well.
- **Feeding:** Apply a balanced, organic fertilizer at the beginning of the growing season to support root development.
- **Pruning and Maintenance:** Snip off dead flowers and trim back excessive growth to maintain plant health and vigor.
- **Pest and Disease Management:** Monitor for common garden pests and fungal diseases. Treat with organic pesticides or fungicides as necessary, and ensure good air circulation to prevent disease.
- **Overwintering:** In colder climates, mulch around the base of the plant to protect the roots from freezing temperatures.
- **Propagation:** Propagate wild yam by dividing the tubers in early spring or late fall, ensuring each piece has at least one growth eye.
- **Harvesting:** The roots of wild yam can be harvested in the fall, after several years of growth, when they are well-developed and contain optimal levels of active compounds.
- **Climate Considerations:** Wild yam thrives in temperate climates with well-defined seasons and prefers a balance of sun and shade, with adequate moisture throughout the growing season.

How to Use Wild Yam

Herbal Teas or Infusions: Wild yam root is cut into small pieces and soaked in boiling water to create an infusion, commonly used to help with digestive discomfort and to balance hormones.

Tinctures: The root of wild yam is often soaked in alcohol to extract its active components, creating a tincture that is used to alleviate menstrual cramps and hormonal imbalances.

Decoctions: A strong decoction is made by simmering the root for an extended period, used for its anti-inflammatory and antispasmodic properties.

Powders: Dried wild yam root can be ground into a powder and used in capsules or mixed with other substances to aid in hormone balance and digestive health.

Ease to Grow: 3-6, Medium Maintenance

Wild Yam is moderately easy to grow, with some attention needed for proper soil conditions and spacing to accommodate its growth habit.

Witch Hazel

Known scientifically as Hamamelis Virginiana, is a small, deciduous tree or shrub native to North America. Renowned for its astringent properties (restricts or tightens tissues), derived from its leaves and bark, which contain tannins and other bioactive compounds. Witch Hazel is traditionally used to soothe skin irritations, reduce inflammation, and help heal minor wounds. Its extracts are commonly found in topical treatments for acne, bruises, and hemorrhoids. The plant flowers in late fall, with unique, fragrant yellow blooms that are both ornamental and functional in herbal medicine.

Skin and Integumentary System

Skin: Witch Hazel acts as an astringent, tightening the skin and reducing inflammation. It is effective in treating acne, eczema, and other skin conditions.

How to Grow Witch Hazel

- **Selecting the Right Variety:** Hamamelis Virginiana, also known as American Witch Hazel, is most commonly used for its medicinal properties. Plants or seeds can be purchased from nurseries or online. Starting from seeds can be challenging due to their dormancy requirements; thus, buying young plants might be preferable.
- **Best Time to Plant Outdoors:** Plant Witch Hazel in the fall or early spring when the weather is cool, and the plant can establish roots without the stress of extreme temperatures.
- **Spacing Outdoor Plants:** Space plants about 15 to 20 feet apart to allow for their mature size and to ensure good air circulation.
- **Container Use and Soil:** Witch Hazel can be grown in large containers using well-draining soil rich in organic matter. Ensure the container has adequate drainage holes.
- **Sunlight and Location:** Prefers full sun to partial shade, with at least 4 to 6 hours of direct sunlight daily. In very hot climates, afternoon shade is beneficial.
- **Watering:** Keep the soil consistently moist, especially during the first few years of growth. Water deeply once a week during dry periods.
- **Feeding:** Apply a layer of compost or a slow-release fertilizer in the early spring to nourish the plant.

- **Pruning and Maintenance:** Prune in late winter or early spring to remove any dead or crossing branches. Snip off dead flowers to promote healthy plant growth.
- **Pest and Disease Management:** Witch Hazel is generally resistant to pests and diseases, but watch for signs of aphids or scale insects and treat with horticultural oils or insecticidal soap if necessary.
- **Overwintering:** No special care is needed for overwintering in its hardiness zones; it is quite frost-resistant.
- **Propagation:** Propagate by seed or softwood cuttings taken in late spring or early summer. Seeds require stratification to break dormancy.
- **Harvesting:** The leaves and bark are harvested in the fall. Leaves are picked when green and vibrant, while bark is stripped from the branches or trunk.
- **Climate Considerations:** Thrives in temperate climates with well-defined seasons, prefers areas with cold winters and warm, not hot, summers.

How to Use Witch Hazel

Tinctures: Witch Hazel bark and leaves are soaked in alcohol to create a tincture, used for its astringent properties to tone skin and reduce inflammation.

Salves-Topical Applications: Extracts from the plant are used in salves, creams, or ointments for soothing skin irritations, healing minor cuts, and reducing inflammation.

Decoctions: A decoction made from the bark can be applied topically for its astringent properties, helping to treat skin issues like acne, bruises, and hemorrhoids.

Compresses: Soaked pads or cloths in Witch Hazel extract are beneficially applied to the skin to soothe burns, wounds, and reduce swelling.

Ease to Grow: 2-5, Low Maintenance
Witch Hazel is relatively easy to grow, tolerating a range of conditions and requiring minimal maintenance once established.

Yarrow

Achillea Millefolium, is a perennial herb with a long history of use in traditional medicine. It is recognized by its feathery leaves and clusters of small, white to pink flowers. Yarrow is valued for its anti-inflammatory, antiseptic, and astringent properties (causes contraction or tightening of tissues). It's been used to treat wounds, reduce fever, and improve circulation. Yarrow contains active compounds such as flavonoids and terpenes, which contribute to its therapeutic effects. Yarrow is also known for supporting digestion and relieving respiratory conditions.

Digestive System
Stomach: Yarrow is used to stimulate appetite and aid digestion by increasing saliva and stomach acid production, easing digestive discomfort and helping to relieve symptoms like indigestion and bloating.

Respiratory System

Lungs: Acts as an expectorant, loosening phlegm in the respiratory tract, thereby easing congestion and facilitating easier breathing, making it beneficial for treating colds and flu.

Cardiovascular System

Blood vessels: Yarrow can improve circulation by dilating blood vessels, which helps to promote blood flow and reduce blood pressure, potentially benefiting cardiovascular health.

Skin and Integumentary System

Skin: Known for its astringent properties, yarrow is effective in treating skin wounds and abrasions. It promotes healing, reduces inflammation, and can help to stop bleeding, making it a valuable herb for topical use on cuts and bruises.

Immune System

General immunity: By stimulating the immune system, yarrow helps the body to combat infections and diseases more effectively. Its bioactive compounds can enhance the body's natural defense mechanisms against pathogens.

How to Grow Yarrow

- **Selecting the Right Variety:** Achillea Millefolium, commonly known as Yarrow, has several varieties with different flower colors ranging from white to pink and yellow. It can be grown from both seeds and starts. Seeds are more readily available and can be sown directly in the garden or started indoors. You can purchase them from garden centers or online seed suppliers.

- **Best Time to Plant Outdoors:** The best time to plant Yarrow is in the spring or fall, allowing the plant to establish itself during mild weather conditions.
- **Spacing Outdoor Plants:** Space Yarrow plants about 1 to 2 feet apart to ensure they have enough room to spread and receive adequate air circulation.
- **Container Use and Soil:** Yarrow grows well in containers using well-draining soil. It prefers a sandy or loamy soil and can tolerate poor soil conditions.
- **Sunlight and Location:** Yarrow thrives in full sun, needing at least 6 hours of direct sunlight daily. It can tolerate partial shade but blooms best in full sun.
- **Watering:** Once established, Yarrow is drought-tolerant and requires minimal watering, but during the initial growth phase, keep the soil evenly moist.
- **Feeding:** Yarrow does not require frequent fertilization. A light application of compost or all-purpose fertilizer in the spring is sufficient.
- **Pruning and Maintenance:** Regularly snip off dead flowers to encourage new growth and prevent the plant from seeding too aggressively.
- **Pest and Disease Management:** Yarrow is relatively resistant to pests and diseases, but it can be susceptible to powdery mildew and rust. Ensure good air circulation and treat with appropriate fungicides if necessary.
- **Overwintering:** Yarrow is hardy and overwinters well without special care in most climates. In very cold regions, a layer of mulch can help protect the roots.
- **Propagation:** Propagate Yarrow by dividing the clumps in the spring or fall or by sowing seeds directly in the garden.

- **Harvesting:** The aerial parts of Yarrow, including leaves and flowers, can be harvested in the summer when the plant is in bloom. They are used fresh or dried for medicinal purposes.
- **Climate Considerations:** Yarrow is adaptable to various climates but grows best in temperate regions. It can tolerate a range of temperatures and weather conditions.

How to Use Yarrow

Herbal Teas or Infusions: Yarrow leaves and flowers are cut and soaked in hot water to make a tea that is used for its anti-inflammatory and digestive benefits.

Tinctures: The aerial parts of yarrow are soaked in alcohol to create a tincture, used to relieve digestive issues, reduce inflammation, and help with wound healing.

Salves-Topical Applications: Yarrow can be infused into creams or ointments to make salves for topical application on wounds, cuts, and skin irritations, utilizing its astringent and healing properties.

Decoctions: A decoction of yarrow is made by boiling the plant parts to concentrate its active compounds, used for its anti-inflammatory and antiseptic benefits.

Powders: Dried yarrow is ground into a powder, which can be used internally for digestive issues or externally as a dusting powder for wounds and skin irritations.

Ease to Grow: 1-3, Low Maintenance

Yarrow is very easy to grow, requiring minimal care, and is highly adaptable to various environmental conditions.

Yucca

A type of plant that you often see in dry areas of the Americas, known for its sturdy, pointed leaves and clusters of white flowers. People have used yucca for health reasons, especially in Native American traditional medicine. This plant has special ingredients like saponins, which can fight inflammation and protect against damage from free radicals. Yucca is good for treating several health problems, including joint pain, skin issues, and stomach problems.

Digestive System

Stomach: Yucca is known to help calm inflammation in the stomach, which can help prevent and heal stomach ulcers. It's thought to coat the stomach lining, protecting it from irritation.

Skin and Integumentary System

Skin: Yucca can be good for the skin because its saponins reduce swelling and redness. This makes it useful for healing skin problems like scratches, rashes, and ulcers, by soothing the skin and reducing irritation.

Musculoskeletal System

Joints: The anti-inflammatory effects of yucca are helpful for easing joint pain and stiffness, which is why it's often used by people with arthritis to reduce their discomfort and improve movement.

How to Grow Yucca

- **Selecting the Right Variety:** Yucca includes several species like Yucca Filamentosa and Yucca Gloriosa, all known for their hardiness and ornamental value. They can be grown from seeds or purchased as young plants from garden centers or online nurseries. Seeds may take longer to germinate, so starts are preferable for quicker results.
- **Best Time to Plant Outdoors:** The ideal planting time is in the spring or early summer, allowing the plant to establish before colder weather.
- **Spacing Outdoor Plants:** Space yucca plants about 3 to 6 feet apart, depending on the species, to accommodate their spread and height.
- **Container Use and Soil:** Yucca plants thrive in containers with well-draining soil, preferably a mix of sand, perlite, and potting soil, to mimic their natural arid environment.
- **Sunlight and Location:** They need full sun, at least 6 to 8 hours daily. Yucca plants can tolerate some light shade but prefer direct sunlight to thrive.
- **Watering:** Yucca plants are drought-tolerant and require minimal watering. Water them deeply but infrequently, allowing the soil to dry out between waterings.
- **Feeding:** Apply a low-nitrogen, slow-release fertilizer once a year in the spring to support growth without promoting excessive foliage.
- **Pruning and Maintenance:** Snip off dead flowers and trim any damaged or dying leaves to keep the plant healthy and tidy.

- **Pest and Disease Management:** Monitor for signs of scale insects or root rot. Treat scale with insecticidal soap and ensure good drainage to prevent root rot.
- **Overwintering:** Most yucca species are frost-resistant. In very cold climates, protect the base of the plant with mulch to insulate the roots.
- **Propagation:** Propagate yucca through division or by planting offsets in the spring or summer.
- **Harvesting:** The flowers, seeds, and sometimes leaves of yucca can be harvested when mature, typically in the late summer or fall. The parts are used for culinary or medicinal purposes.
- **Climate Considerations:** Yucca plants are best suited for arid to semi-arid climates, thriving in areas with low rainfall and high temperatures. They can withstand some cold but prefer a dry, warm climate.

How to Use Yucca

Herbal Teas or Infusions: The flowers of the yucca plant are sometimes soaked in hot water to create an herbal tea, which is consumed for its potential health benefits, including antioxidants.
Tinctures: Yucca root can be used to make a tincture, which is believed to have anti-inflammatory and pain-relieving properties.
Decoctions: The roots of yucca can be boiled to make a strong decoction, often used traditionally to treat joint pain and inflammation.
Culinary Uses: Yucca flowers and stems are edible and can be cooked and eaten. The flowers are sometimes added to salads, while the stems are cooked similarly to asparagus.

Ease to Grow: 2-3, Low Maintenance

Yucca is an easy-to-grow plant, thriving in well-draining soil with full sun exposure and requiring minimal water, making it suitable for xeriscaping (a landscaping approach that focuses on water conservation and uses drought-resistant plants) or arid garden designs.

Glossary of Terms

Adaptogenic - Adaptogens are herbs that help the body adapt to stress, supporting overall well-being and resilience. They regulate physiological processes and promote balance, enhancing the body's natural resistance to stressors.

Annuals - Annual herbs complete their entire life cycle, from seed germination to seed production and termination, within one growing season, typically dying after flowering.

Antispasmodic - Herbs that relax and relieve muscle spasms and cramps, easing discomfort. They work by calming nerve impulses and promoting smooth muscle function, offering relief for various conditions like digestive issues.

Anxiolytic Properties - Herbs have calming effects, reducing anxiety and promoting relaxation. They work by regulating neurotransmitters in the brain, providing relief from stress and anxiety-related symptoms.

Astringent Properties - Astringent herbs have a contracting effect, tightening tissues and reducing secretions. They are used topically to tone skin and internally to help control diarrhea and support digestive health.

Atherosclerosis - A condition where plaque builds up in arteries, narrowing and hardening them. Herbs like garlic and hawthorn may help manage atherosclerosis by supporting cardiovascular health.

Biennial - A biennial herb completes its life cycle in two years. In the first year, it grows leaves, stems, and roots, and in the second, it flowers, produces seeds, and then dies.

Carminative Properties - Refer to an herb's ability to relieve digestive gas, reduce bloating, and alleviate stomach discomfort. Herbs with these properties can soothe the digestive tract and improve digestion.

Corms - In herbal medicine, corms are short, vertical, swollen underground plant stems that store nutrients. They serve as a storage organ and a means for vegetative reproduction.

Deciduous - Refers to plants that shed their leaves annually, usually in response to seasonal changes, allowing them to conserve energy during adverse conditions.

Mediterranean Climate - Characterized by mild, wet winters and hot, dry summers. It supports the growth of a diverse range of herbs known for their aromatic flavors and therapeutic properties.

Neem Oil - Neem oil, derived from the neem tree, possesses antibacterial, antifungal, and anti-inflammatory properties. It's used in herbal medicine to treat skin conditions, repel pests, and improve dental health.

Perennial - Plants that live for more than two years. They grow back each spring from their root system, providing a continuous harvest for culinary or medicinal uses.

Rhizomes - Underground stems that grow horizontally, found in some herbs. They store nutrients, help in vegetative reproduction, and can have medicinal properties, like anti-inflammatory effects.

Stratification - A process of treating seeds to simulate natural conditions they must experience before germination, often involving cold and moist exposure, crucial for breaking seed dormancy in many herbal species.

Woody - In herbal medicine, "woody" describes plants with hard, fibrous tissues in stems, roots, and branches, often found in perennials, shrubs, and trees, providing structural support and longevity.

Xeriscaping - Involves designing gardens and landscapes to reduce water usage, using drought-resistant herbs and plants to create sustainable, low-maintenance herbal gardens.

♡ Thank You ♡

Did you enjoy this book?

Your feedback helps us provide the best quality books and helps other readers like you discover healthy helpful books as well.

It would mean so much to me and our lush grove family, if you wouldn't mind taking two minutes to share your thoughts, as an actual posted review wherever you purchased this book.

I personally read and truly treasure every comment as a source of personal inspiration and encouragement.

Join Our Lush Grove Community

Unlock Exclusive Content
Choose your FREE welcome gift!

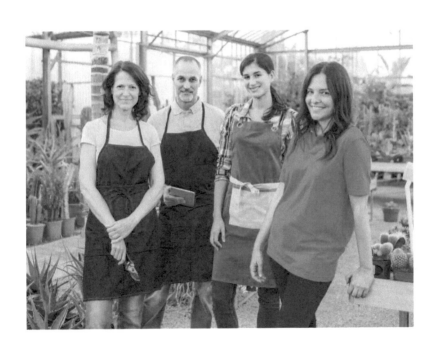

Made in United States
Troutdale, OR
06/04/2024

20296342R20246